Happiness and Fulfilment in Dentistry

D1563415

This book is dedicated to
my wife Kay

*"A good wife is surely the finest jewel
a man can possess"*

Happiness and Fulfilment in Dentistry

Peter Glazebrook

Foreword by
Peter E. Dawson

LONDON
Quintessence Publishing Company Limited

© 1985 Peter Glazebrook

First published 1985 by
Quintessence Publishing Company Limited,
36 Canbury Park Road, Kingston-upon-Thames
Surrey KT2 6JX, England

ISBN 1 85097 002 5

Typeset by Alacrity Phototypesetters,
Banwell Castle, Weston-super-Mare
Printed in Great Britain by
Biddles Ltd, Guildford, Surrey

Contents

Foreword

Those of us who have practiced dentistry for twenty-five years or more have witnessed some remarkable advances in both technique and understanding of virtually every aspect of dental diagnosis and treatment. A high percentage of the procedures we use today in our practices utilize methods and materials that were not even heard of when I was in dental school . . . and with proper treatment, we have achieved a truly impressive capability to treat even more complex problems with predictable success. The state of the art and science of dentistry has reached a level of sophistication that makes it possible for any dentist to give his patients optimum oral health, comfort and natural aesthetic beauty.

Unfortunately, while great advances were being made in preventive dentistry and treatment capabilities, there were counter forces at work to prevent patients from having the level of dental care that was possible. Some of these forces were political . . . and while it is painfully obvious that the great socialistic attempt to standardize fees and services resulted in lowering the quality of treatment . . . it should also be obvious that professional conduct would not allow that to happen without a change in moral and ethical standards.

True professionalism, especially in a health service, requires that we use our education and our reasoning skills within a professional atmosphere of discipline, honesty and hard work to provide the best treatment we can give.

It is true that we often have constraints imposed because of health, patient desire, intelligence and finances, but these are factors that must be thoughtfully evaluated when deciding what is best for the patient.

We can't dictate values, but we can examine the consequences of values and it is obvious that when ethics is reduced to merely taking advantage of 'the system', we end up with no ethics at all. Don't worry about whether you are serving your fellow man ... just milk the system and let the patient beware.

Why do I bring up such topics as ethics, and morality in this foreword? Because I firmly believe that the lack of a general moral perspective will be the cause of the greatest polarization that our profession has ever known. All the technical expertise in the world will fail if the 'New Morality' gives too little credence to honesty, to discipline, and to integrity.

We have been fortunate in our people serving profession of dentistry. We have had many true professionals who have clearly declared that we owe our patients the best care, skill and judgement that we can logically give them.

There are many pressures being exerted on practitioners today ... pressures to forego the old ethical standards, not just through social legislation, but also in favour of high volume, advertising, or other forms of opportunism that are the antithesis of quality, caring service. This is now and will continue to be at the one end of the polarization we mentioned. I believe dentists who chose this path will be more unhappy, more unfulfilled, and less rewarded than any dentists in history.

But what about the other side ... I believe the dentist who truly cares enough for his patients to master his skills and provide optimal treatment in a caring atmosphere will find more reward, more fulfilment, more true enjoyment in practice than dentists have ever experienced.

Many dentists have had the wonderful good fortune of having a role model in the search for a philosophy of practice. Even though the problems and the influences of today are different, the principles of this philosophy are more valid than ever. Furthermore these principles will not only serve as a guide to successful practice, they are a blueprint for a successful, rewarding, happy life. Of course I am referring to the philosophy of Dr. L.D. Pankey.

To know Dr. Pankey is to know his principles work. He is successful by every standard of measurement. He is admired and loved by his patients and his peers. He is a happy, fulfilled person who continues to give unselfishly. He simply practices what he has preached, and obviously it works. It is doubtful if anyone in our time has influenced dentistry and dentists more than L.D. Pankey. His contributions in the technical aspects of dentistry are in themselves noteworthy. His role as a motivator has caused thousands of dentists to upgrade their goals and strive to do more complete dentistry for their patients. He has been a catalyst for bringing great minds together in synergistic efforts to distil out the practical from the experimental, and in the process has stimulated uncounted others to be better than they would have been if they had never met this man.

Many people are not aware that the L.D. Pankey Institute for Advanced Dental Education was not founded by Dr. Pankey. Rather it was founded by many of the dentists he had helped ... as a tribute to him. Its purpose was and is to close the gap between what is known and what is being practiced. I can say without reservation, that the dentists who have taken full advantage of the Institute and who have followed the philosophy in their lives, are among the finest dentists in the world ... but just as important, they are happy. They are fulfilled and hopefully they are the guardians of professionalism for the future.

Dentistry has needed this book. The philosophy has too often been misunderstood because only portions of it were heard. For the philosophy to be valid, it must be complete. The author has not missed any of the pertinent parts and anyone who studies this treatise will benefit to the degree the concept is accepted.

Please remember though that this is a dynamic philosophy ... it is a never ending search for excellence and understanding. That is why Dr. Pankey is still excited and enthusiastic with dentistry and with life in his eighth decade ... and you can be, too.

Peter E. Dawson

Preface

No man is an island unto himself, and knowledge transcends all ages and frontiers. Every philosopher in the world has taken ideas freely from others, developed them and incorporated them into his own thinking. This is no different and I have taken ideas from many sources to weave together in this philosophy.

I have gleaned these ideas over half a century of life, from my parents, and schoolteachers, from my wife Kay and her parents, and from books, ministers of religion of various creeds, and from many other fine people in the world. But the most powerful impact on my mind has come from two of the greatest people I have ever met in any profession, Dr. L.D. Pankey and Dr. Loren Miller. I am happy and privileged to call these men my friends.

Over many years I had thought out my philosophy of life and tried to apply it to my profession. It was hard going and I frequently felt that I was 'the only one in step', not realising how many other dentists were tramping the same solitary road. And then I went to the Pankey Institute.

I shall never forget my first morning there: a strange country, a strange hotel, and by the time I found my way about I was late for the traditional breakfast and somewhat embarrassed. I need not have been. A man rose from the top table and came to greet me with an outstretched hand and a smile which said 'love' and 'welcome' more eloquently than a thousand words. He introduced himself as Loren Miller, and I warmed to him from the beginning, little realising just how high my opinion of this man was to rise. Later we had lectures on philosophy from him. I could hardly believe my ears. He was speaking my own mind and my own thoughts, but going much further than my thinking had gone, and all was collated into a marvellously whole, rounded philosophy. I knew that I was home, and that the hard work of thinking over the next twenty five years had largely been done for me. It was one of the most stimulating experiences of my whole life.

It is this collation of philosophy which I seek to present in this work: the thinking of Dr. L.D. Pankey, as expounded by himself and by Loren Miller, all woven into my own thoughts. How lucky we are to have people of such stature gracing our profession! To them I wish I could say more than 'thank you'. And it is from this wish and as a tribute to them that this book has been written. But, though these are the words of L.D. and Loren as interpreted by me, since I am the writer I must take full responsibility for them. Nevertheless, without 'L.D.' and Loren, this work would never have been written, and it has been written in an endeavour to help others to understand the fullness of joy and happiness and achievement which can come from the practice of dentistry, as expounded by great men, and as experienced by many of the finest dentists in the world. Dentists, from the most renowned such as Pete Dawson or Alvin Fillastre, through to many local dentists working on main streets in small towns all over the world, have proved in their own practice the truth of the Pankey ideal. May the reader be helped to experience a similar uplift in quality of life from reading these words in this book.

In addition to these two 'greats' already mentioned, there are many others whom I must acknowledge for their contribution to 'my' philosophy. Firstly my father (one of the few, very few, practising British dentists who did not join the health service in 1948). Only a dentist's son can really appreciate the tremendous advantage of being 'born into the profession'. So much is absorbed just by seeing what goes on in the laboratory, and hearing the gist of general conversation and 'shop talk'. My father also set me an admirable example of striving for excellence in operative work and the importance of service to the patients, as well as the ideal of fine fee for service dentistry. All this on top of putting me through dental school. It was a truly firm base to work on.

Then there are my teachers at dental school, principally Jimmy Mansie, 'my' consultant tutor, who taught me so much, frequently throwing me in at the deep end. And Ronnie Emslie, the young registrar, always looking for ways to stick the gum back on to the tooth. They gave me a vision of daring to the utmost of my knowledge and ability and beyond, and not being content with the limits set by teachers.

At East Grinstead and Mount Vernon, there was the example of surgery done by Terry Ward and Paul Toller. Such consummate operators! More recently are the famous men who have influenced me in the field of occlusion: Niles Guichet and Arnie Lauritzen. A great many dentists, renowned today in their own right, owe so much to these two; and also to Peter K. Thomas, one of the most able and energetic apostles of good dentistry, along with that other 'great' of the West coast, Charles Stuart, a legend in his own time.

Then — and extremely important indeed — there are the dentists associated with the Pankey Institute, John Anderson, Henry Tanner, Jim Potts, Alvin Fillastre, and above all, Pete Dawson. The Pankey approach is to my mind the most logical and straightforward approach to occlusion, and of all the teachers, there is none like Pete Dawson for clear thinking, simply expressed. His understanding is basic, and I unhesitatingly recommend his lectures and his book[1] to any young aspiring dental surgeon. All the 'Pankey' lecturers deliver their teaching on dentistry in a package of people-orientated dentistry, and this is one of the major attractions of the 'Pankey School'. It doesn't just concern itself with clinical affairs, but puts all things in a human context.

I must thank Gerry Banks, a padre in the army in Malaya, for teaching me the 'meaning of philosophy' back in 1950 and '51, when we sat up through the night as radio 'hams' waiting for the next CQ20 contact.

Lastly, my incomparable wife Kay, who has not only borne with me whilst writing the book but who has been a constant source of inspiration through living out her life and our life to such high standards in our marriage. Truly, a good wife is the finest jewel any man can possess.

Peter Glazebrook

✦ 1 ✦

The Path to Happiness

Why are so many dentists unhappy? A survey carried out in the United States showed that about one third of the dentists questioned would *most probably* not choose dentistry if they could start their careers again, and a further one third of the dentists would *definitely* choose something else. This means that only one third of dentists were satisfied with their choice of career, and of these the number that was really fulfilled was very much smaller. Experience in Britain would suggest similar proportions here. This is a tragedy; particularly since dentistry is potentially one of the most fulfilling and satisfying professions.

Why do so many dentists fail to find satisfaction in their work?

It is in an attempt to answer this question that this book has been written. It is intended to help dentists of all ages to achieve fulfilment and satisfaction in their careers and in their lives.

Everything in this life (including success) must be paid for. The dentist who would succeed must be prepared to study and to understand. Both are extremely demanding, involving the hardest work of all, thinking. To paraphrase George Bernard Shaw — about two percent of people think, another two or three percent like to think that they think, and the rest would rather die than think. So the aspiring dentist must put himself in the top two percent of people and use his brains if he would achieve the manifold rewards which are there for the taking in dentistry. In short, he must become a philosopher.

Philosophy used to be the basis of all university curricula, but it has become rather unfashionable today. It is considered to be something reserved for the triple A grade academic. As a result, the rest of us are never taught how to string our thoughts together, and we become creatures of opinion. The problem with having opinions is that there is no pressure on us to study our opinions as they relate to each other, with the result that we often unwittingly hold contradictory opinions on different subjects. This could be seen to be so if only we would look at them together. Our prejudices and our laziness contrive to make sure we do not examine our opinions carefully, because then we might have to do something about our dual standards. That would mean leaving our comfortable cosy niche. So we remain opinionated and this becomes like a ball and chain which stops us from progressing in life.

We can all try to become philosophers. A philosophy is a complete system, in which all ideas and opinions are related in a harmonious whole. It is like a jig-saw puzzle in which all the pieces fit together to form a beautiful picture. The picture does not emerge in all its beauty and harmony until all the pieces have been set in their proper place, and an attempt to introduce pieces from another jig-saw puzzle would only spoil the fit and the harmony. Similarly in our lives; if we live by a true philosophy then the complete picture of our lives will be beautiful and satisfying. If we live by opinions, then we are just an ugly pile of unrelated bits and pieces, not really knowing who we are, or where we are going in this life. So this book advocates a philosophy. But do not be put off by that. Philosophy is extremely satisfying, designed to provoke thought, and anything that provokes constructive thought is good. Even if one disagrees with the views expressed, one should think out why one disagrees, and whether in the end the disagreement is justified or not. Of course such disagreement may dictate a change of opinion; and pride can make this a very difficult thing to do. But it is never impossible, and once one can begin to change, and understand the whole picture, then one's philosophy becomes one of the most exciting discoveries of one's life. Suddenly everything fits together and the way ahead becomes clear and inviting; life becomes meaningful, and in Loren Miller's favourite phrase, one can begin to soar.

But having a philosophy is much easier if one has a frame on which to hang it. It is like having strong girders bolted together to form the framework of a building: so that the bricks needed to complete the building can then be neatly put in their proper place. I am greatly indebted to that very fine dentist and most admirable person, Dr. L.D. Pankey for showing me a framework on which to build my philosophy, and I hope that an understanding of the ideas he has given me will help the reader to marshall his thoughts and build up his (or her) own philosophy of life. And this is the crucial point. The philosophy must end up by being a *personal* philosophy; not my philosophy or L.D. Pankey's philosophy, or Loren Miller's philosophy, but yours. You have to own it; to be able to call it your very own.

Dr. Pankey's Philosophy

What then is Pankey's philosophy? The basic idea is not new, in fact it is well over two thousand years old. Our first record of the idea is from the writings of Aristotle, but he may well have developed his thoughts from those of his contemporaries. Dr. Pankey calls Aristotle's framework the Cross of Life and its basic principle is that if one wants to be happy then one has to keep one's life in balance. Whenever we get our lives out of balance, it is because we are neglecting one or more of the important ingredients of life, by concentrating too much time and energy on just one aspect of living. This leads to a completely unbalanced personality and life style, and although we might well succeed in that part of living on which we are concentrating our main effort, the riches and treasures of the other parts of life can be withering and dying. The result of this is that we will not be fulfilled, and when the success we have been striving for comes our way, it will be hollow and empty, and will seem worthless, because there will be nothing else in life to have been successful for. Who does not know of the rich man who is lonely because he neglected his family in the 'push for the top'?

Cross of Life and the Cross of Reward

According to Aristotle, the main things in life are Work, Play, Love and Worship. If we would be happy, we must continually devote an appropriate amount of time and energy to those four bastions of living and fulfilment. These can be shown pictorially as a cross, with happiness at the centre.

```
                    WORK
                     |
LOVE ——————————  HAPPINESS  ———————— WORSHIP
                     |
                    PLAY
```

The main part of this book will look at these four aspects of life in individual detail, and the chapters of the thesis correspond to them. But I wish to emphasize that it is important to maintain the overall idea of the principle of balance whilst reading them. Do not get so close to the trees that you cannot appreciate the wood as a whole.

Dr. Pankey was not content to leave things there. We are dentists and must work out our salvation against the background of our profession. For this reason, he designed another cross, which he called *the cross of reward*. This cross is related directly to dentistry, but can easily be adapted to relate to any other profession or calling. It is based on the achievement of adequate rewards in professional life, and the rewards we seek are of two kinds, both denoted by the letter S. The first S stands for spiritual rewards. If we are to be happy, we must feel that we are constructive members of society and are doing noble and worthwhile work. We must be proud of our accomplishments and hold our heads up high, knowing we are achieving what we set out to do, on the highest professional and ethical level.

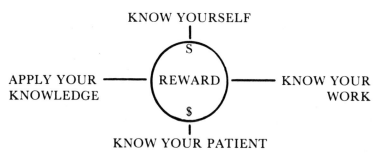

The main object of Dr. Pankey's four arms of the cross of reward is to achieve Fulfilment. The names of the arms are KNOW YOURSELF, KNOW YOUR PATIENT, KNOW YOUR WORK, and APPLY YOUR KNOW-LEDGE. If we understand these four things and put them into practice, we will not only reap the spiritual rewards, but will also reap the reward denoted by the second S, which has two lines drawn through it $ so. This leads to fulfilment. One aims to be financially successful, whilst ensuring money does not become one's god. G od management of money is necessary to avoid failure; but the financial rewards will flow all the more readily if one has sorted out the spiritual side of one's approach to work. If we do know ourselves and just what we do have to offer, know our patients and what they desire to achieve through their dentistry, then we can begin to apply our knowledge in the most meaningful way, and the more we know about our work the more knowledge we will be able to apply.

If all this is done by a practitioner properly motivated, the patient will realise that everything recommended is for his well-being. And when he knows that he is also getting a very high order of expertise, he will be truly grateful. He will appreciate good dentistry and will tell his friends. Success for the dentist will be assured. Man has not changed over the millenia. He who really does offer a full measure and running over, is still a rarity, and is still the most sought after of his kind, whatever his particular calling. Good service and value are never out of date.

Once again it is worth emphasizing the principle of balance. All aspects of this 'cross of rewards' must be applied in balance before the rewards become apparent. I know good dentists who have a very high standard of knowledge and operative technique, but who are relatively unsuccessful. This is often because they do not know their patient and cannot offer relevant treatment to a particular person. Sometimes, it is because they do not know themselves, and have not overcome their own weaknesses. Some may have a very good knowledge of their work but find it difficult to pluck up the confidence to apply that knowledge in more difficult cases.

It must be stressed that this second cross cannot be looked at separately from the 'Cross of Life'. Both must be considered and applied in proper relation to each other. Remember we are following a philosophy not just a collection of opinions. The relaxed and loving attitude of mind that comes from a full understanding of the cross of life is a wonderful builder of confidence for the patient and therefore a fine practice builder. There is no analgesic in the world half as effective as a good chairside manner.

Good Health

Good health is important, if one is to be successful and fulfilled in one's career. We cannot function if we are flat on our backs from some physical ailment, and even minor physical disabilities can cripple our performance at the chairside.

Dentistry is an extremely demanding profession and we need to be in tip top condition if we are to cope with the demands it makes on us, both mental and physical. Mental and physical health are not the only kinds of well being. What about our financial health, and the health of our practices and of our own dental health? It has been said that the dentist's dental condition is a mirror of his own attitude towards his profession. We all ought to ask ourselves, 'Am I a good example of fine dentistry?' And if we are not, what right have we to recommend patients treatment we do not countenance in our own mouths!

Thus Dr. Pankey evolved his cross of good health, although he described it this time as a four legged stool, because our health *is* our support. And like success and fulfilment, good health is not just luck; it can be worked for and we can avoid a good deal of ill health if we plan our lives (with a little discipline) along the lines of preventive medicine. We can make our bodies more resistant to disease, and maintain our physical abilities by good diet and prudent physical exercise, suitable to our age and personalities. Dr. Pankey himself is a shining example of this. He walks three miles every morning, at almost racing speed, and every mile he jogs for 250 yards. Not bad for a man of 82 years, and keeping up with him is no mean feat as I can testify from personal experience.

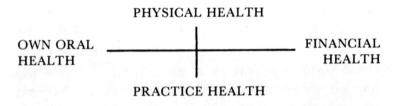

PHYSICAL HEALTH

OWN ORAL HEALTH — FINANCIAL HEALTH

PRACTICE HEALTH

The philosophy of good health must, of course, be related to the other demands of life. It is no use becoming a hypochondriac. There is no need to spend all your spare time on sport, ignoring everything else. But it is so easy to go to the opposite extreme and spend all one's efforts trying to build up a business, and forget all about health in the meanwhile.

The separate headings will be considered in detail later on, but it is apposite to remark here that it is difficult to run any business when the finance is not properly thought out. Financial worries are very real and can not only cause disaster in business but can severely affect one's general health and mental attitude. It is very debilitating to try to work in a disorganised establishment, where there are tensions and emotional upsets which may affect principal, staff and patients. Conversely, it is a pleasure to work in a well run, healthy practice. Such considerations are implied in the first two crosses. Know yourself, think how your attitude can affect the health of your patients, and realise how your patients will be affected by the atmosphere in your practice. This will affect the level of your success and fulfilment.

Finally, we must remember that Rome was not built in a day. A philosophy cannot be achieved overnight and it is important to realise one has to think and work at it, and above all to hasten forward slowly. Have a sensible plan, and try not to introduce new ideas into the practice until the implications are fully understood. Persevere, and have a positive attitude of mind. Think success, think fulfilment, and as you become steeped in such ideas they may be achieved in your life. You can have a practice in which you work the hours you want to work, in the place you want to be, in the atmosphere you delight in, and with the financial and spiritual rewards which fulfil all your desires. Good Luck.

2

Know Yourself

A philosopher, any philosopher, must know himself (or herself). This is the most important first step. It involves knowing one's weaknesses and one's strengths; where one is and where one wants to be; what one has achieved, and what one wants to achieve. These things are so important, yet the majority of us hardly give them a second thought. The power of positive thought is tremendous. What the mind can conceive and believe, it can achieve.

But most of us achieve very little! Why? Because too many of us are alert to our limitations, but scarcely aware of our strengths. We lack the vision to change things. We are all too ready to accept our situation and our weaknesses as limits, and our strengths as only what we have been using so far. Most of us reach little more than ten percent of our potential.

Again, why? We accept things because we have been conditioned to do so, or rather because we have not seen ourselves as achievers. All of us are the product of heredity and environment. We all inherit basic characteristics from our parents in our genetic structure, not only physical attributes like height and colour of eyes, but mental abilities like a capacity for logical thought. A slow mental plodder will never be a quick witted mercurial type of person, and there is no point wishing otherwise. Unfortunately, we all do go through a phase of wishing we were someone else, or at least valuing another's qualities above our own. But this sort of envy is the road to unhappiness, and the sooner we recognise the advantages of our own basic make up, the better for us. Then we can do the important thing, which is to realise our own uniqueness, make ourselves into the best of our type of person and to use our good points to advantage.

In order to do this, it is then necessary to understand the effect of environment upon us and our way of thinking. Think of yourself as a little mouse in the corner and that is what you will become. Think of yourself as violent and you will become so, possibly ending up as a terrorist or a criminal. And the same applies to success and failure. You have to think success in order to achieve success. But in order to think for oneself at all, one has to come to terms with the effect of environment on the mind and personality.

Growing Up

Our minds are like computers. They are programmed by all the information fed into them over our formative years. The initial programming is extremely strong and very basic. It is difficult to eradicate or change, but *not* impossible. The Chinese, who invented paper, have another way of putting this. They say that one's life is like a sheet of paper, and everyone that one meets writes something on it. Of course, we write on other people's pieces of paper too, and the attitude of the societies in which we live is the sum of the effect which we all have on each other. The boldest writing is that which was written in our childhood.

The first people to write on our sheet of paper are our

parents, and the process begins when the child is still in the womb. Pain can be felt, the mother's emotions sensed and noises heard. When the child is born it is soon subjected to more, and deeper, experiences. Usually, though unfortunately not always, it experiences a mother's love; it learns to talk and to walk, to make its wishes known, and how to respond to others. In all this the parents, particularly the mother, play a major part.

This programming, for good or bad, goes on through the whole of one's early life, and at first we can do little about it. We are under the control of our parents, who do all the writing on our paper. Then nannies, relatives, and school teachers. This continues until puberty, when most children are beginning to observe that the world around them is not all the same as it is at home and in school. By then, or sometimes earlier, most people will have decided that they do not have to let anyone write on their sheet of paper any more; they can decide how they want to programme themselves, and are beginning to have an idea of the sort of person they want to be. The next ten years will probably be devoted to experiencing the world, trying to eradicate that which is not wanted from one's memory banks and sifting and sorting through ideas which could be useful.

The years from 25 to 30 years of age are likely to be a time of consolidation, that of collating one's information and making the firm decisions as to the correct way ahead. Plato said that thirty should be the year of maturity, and he felt people ought not to be expected to be in positions of influence under that age.

Unfortunately, many people do not carry the process through to its conclusion, but get stuck along the line, and remain permanently immature. They tend to blame everything on their parents' supposed failures and use that as an excuse for all their own faults and inadequacies. As if their parents could be perfect! As if anyone could be perfect!

Of course, parents are not perfect, and neither are we. It is up to us to make the best of our early environment and build on that. And if we have not overcome our childhood environment by the time we are thirty, then it is no good looking back and blaming our parents for everything. The fault is ours. We should be the master of our own fate, the captain of our own soul.

Self Knowledge

Once this is understood, we can begin to look at ourselves and find why it is that we are not all that we would like to be. This self knowledge is the key to happiness and has been recognised over thousands of years as it brings with it the virtue of humility. Every virtue has its corresponding 'devil's virtue' which is a cruel parody intended to draw one's mind away from the truth, and the devil seems to have been particularly successful in parodying humility as a cringing lack of self confidence. Nothing could be further from the truth. Humility is positive, and a source of strength. It has two aspects, the appreciation of one's faults, and the appreciation of one's strengths. If anything, the first is the most important and the most positive.

For all of us, our own weakness is our own worst enemy. Our weakness is like a millstone around our necks, preventing us from getting on either spiritually or materially in the world. We do far more damage to ourselves with our own failings than any enemy can ever do. Conversely, if we control and overcome our weaknesses, we become so strong that it almost makes it impossible for our enemies to hurt us. Consider an illustration:

There was a boxer with the best right cross in the world. When he hit the opponent with his right cross, that was the end of the bout, because his adversary was knocked out. The boxer was well aware of his strength of punch, but he also had a weakness, a 'glass jaw' which he refused to admit as important. The result was that in his first two fights he was so confident of his own punch that he omitted to look to his defence, and was knocked out in the first round. At last he realised that he did have a weakness, and asked his coach what to do about it. The coach said he must keep his guard well up and circle away from his opponent's strong punch, and make sure his chin was tucked well down on his chest to form a difficult target. The result was that on the next fight he survived his adversary's attacks, and when he saw his opening in the third round, he brought over his right cross and won by a knockout. It wasn't until he learnt to overcome his own weakness and exercise self discipline that his strong points were of any avail to him at all!

So it is with all of us. And the greatest weakness for us all is our own second rate self image. We are aware of our weaknesses; we under-estimate our strengths, unsure of what to do about either; we drift along through life, accepting the bouquets and brickbats as they come. But we can do something to change ourselves if we want to.

A Plan

Firstly, we need a goal. It is worthwhile first to set a modest goal, one which is well within our capacity to reach in a fairly short time. Then we have to make up our minds that we are going to make the effort needed to achieve it. This is very important, for there is a price to pay for everything in this life. As the sage said, 'Whatever thou want in this world, O discontented man, step up, pay the price, and take it'.

There are two important ideas in this saying. First is the idea of discontentment, the second of being prepared to pay the price. Discontentment has been described as the difference between what we would like to be and the effort necessary to achieve it. The very fact that one would like to be better, either materially or spiritually, is evidence of discontentment. The fact that one is worse than one would like to be is the measure of one's refusal to pay the price of making the effort. And the effort usually means the difficult process of thought, followed by the necessary action to achieve what has been thought about. Coming to terms with our weaknesses must mean self-discipline and that always hurts. But it can be done. So the process must be first setting the goal, then giving a time limit, then deciding what needs to be done, both to eradicate our weakness and to use our strength. A thorough appraisal of both is necessary.

Finally, it is so important to *write all these things down*, then one can look at the writing every month and check one's progress. If it is not written down, then there is all too great a danger that time will slip by with nothing having been achieved.

Once a simple goal has been attained in this manner one can begin to set goals for longer periods, and even for life. Start asking yourself questions. What do you expect out of your business? What do you expect from your marriage and family? What do you want to achieve at home? What do you want from the future in terms of travel, knowledge, artistic appreciation, sport, financial security, spiritual welfare, etc? All these things are vitally important and can be quantified and made to come true if you have a sound attitude of mind, and a positive self image. Ultimately, there is no reason why you should not own your own private jet plane, and have houses and villas scattered around the world *if you want to*. And there is no reason why this cannot be achieved concurrently with having a happy family and a first class spiritual life, provided you have your priorities right and keep all things in balance. But what does it profit a man to gain the whole world and lose his soul? No one truly loves an old recluse of a multi-millionaire. Abraham Maslow,[2] a psychologist of our time, who studied the most mentally healthy and fulfilled people, found that they built on a foundation of basic needs which were satisfied, to achieve a greater and greater satisfaction of the more spiritual things in life; in this way they achieved a greater fulfilment in every sphere of life and became leading lights in their field. We can become leading lights in our own field, professionally or socially if we wish to accept the challenge and set our sights high enough. If we do not accept the challenge then we will forever regret our lost opportunities, and never achieve the maximum happiness possible in this world.

Having appreciated one's uniqueness and tried achieving a simple goal, the way is now open to raise one's sights. But the key is knowledge of ourselves and our uniqueness. We can admire others, but in the end we will achieve most by developing our unique talents and overcoming our unique weaknesses; so pride must be set aside, and we must take an honest look at ourselves.

In particular, we must all look at our circumstances and our temperament. Only then can we set realistic objectives. It is no good for most newly qualified dentists to think about buying an aeroplane or a Rolls Royce immediately, because there will be need for investment in business and then investment in a home, and then providing for family, etc. So whilst the Rolls Royce may be an ultimate goal, a good investment in a dental practice is more important at the moment. And whilst good holidays and party-going may be desirable at a later stage of life, it is important in the early stages to husband one's resources and build up one's marriage and family ties. Again, the type of life one wants can influence the type of practice one goes into and its situation. If you want to live in a warm climate, or in the mountains, then decide which is right for you and do it. Such decisions are not the last word. You may be able to sell up and move elsewhere later if you change your mind.

Spiritual and artistic matters are most important. Are you interested in music, the stage, literature or sport? All these are part of life and one should make an effort to recognise one's unique need and ensure that it is fulfilled.

And in our practices, we have more decisions to make. Do we want to be solo practitioners doing our own thing? Is our temperament such that a partnership would be preferable? If so, what kind of partnership, profit sharing or expense sharing, for example? There are so many variables. Are we more suited to working in a hospital or teaching school, or in the armed forces? All these things must be answered. And how do we set up our practice when we do get cracking, do we do all types of dentistry, or do we decide there are some things we would like to do and others which we would rather delegate? It will all depend on our temperament. And what about our approach to patients? I like my patients to relate to me, but I know one dentist who admits he has a problem with personal relationships, and encourages his patients to relate to his female staff. That's neither good nor bad, it is his solution to his unique problems, which he has understood, and which seems to work well for him. And the fact that his girls are always building him up in the eyes of his patients is good for his positive self image.

Self Image

The idea of a positive self image is so important it bears looking at in greater depth. We *are* worthwhile and our unique characteristics are valuable and important if we make the most of them. This is the clue, be positive, think of yourself as the worthwhile being that you are, and build up this positive side of your nature so that you can be proud of yourself. People don't seem to have changed much over the last six or seven thousand years, and even the story of Adam and Eve is really an attempt to make people realise that everyone is imperfect — we all have a 'fallen nature'. Think what this means: you are not alone, everyone else is inadequate and imperfect too! No one is perfect, and no one can ever be perfect. Therefore the fact that you are not a perfect person or a perfect dentist should not dismay you. All the people who have succeeded in life have done so by overcoming their weakness. They had to strive against their imperfections as you have to. We all have to overcome our inadequacies and work towards perfection, even though perfection is unattainable. This striving for improvement is known as the pursuit of excellence.

The pursuit of excellence is a wonderful thing because it is a journey which lasts a whole life through. There is always something worthwhile to achieve, something exciting to be found out about, something to widen our horizon and our ability. And each one of us can achieve these things in our unique way. We all have enormous power, much more than we appreciate. Most people only use a very small part of their brain power in this life. Just believe in yourself and seek to extend the boundaries of your ability and your knowledge and there is virtually nothing which you cannot achieve. If you have done so much already using only a small percentage of your ability, just think what you can achieve if you really try.

So go out and make the most of yourself. Make a promise to do your utmost and write it down. Then take it out and look at it in a month's time and see what you have done about it. Make your positive commitment now. Remember, the woods would be very silent if only the birds with the best voices sang.

3

Know Your Patient

The patient is a human being, just like the dentist. This means he has fears, frustrations, ambitions, and desires in his own way, just like the dentist. And just like the dentist, he (or she) is unique.

This individuality of the patient, his humanity, may be forgotten by the dentist for most of the time, and this stems from our basic training at dental school. When we were students we had no knowledge of our own and no experience to go on, so we had to be given clinical limits as to how far we could go in our treatment. We were like children who were told not to play outside the field next to the farmhouse, because if we strayed into the woods, the wolf might get us! But this restriction does not last forever, and when we grow up, we are supposed to know how to cope with the animals of the forest. After all, one cannot stay in the home field all one's life. Unfortunately, the teachers in the dental schools become so familiar with the restrictions they place upon the students that they tend to accept them for themselves also, and since academics are the professional establishment in most countries, they end up by setting restrictive standards for the profession as a whole, and dentists generally are constrained to treat their patients within the clinical parameters set down by the academics.

For these reasons, in the majority of cases, dentists tend to treat their patients as clinical specimens. Thus it is assumed for example that bridges can only be made if there is 'X' ratio crown to bony support etc. and no attempt is made to find out if the patient really needs the bridge for personal reasons. And this is the nub, very few patients are ever asked, or allowed to tell their own desires and needs to the dentist; it is hardly surprising therefore that the examination carried out by the dental surgeon is usually confined to the clinical details.

Dentists who so restrict themselves, miss the majority of the joys and satisfactions of dental practice; and their patients frequently fail to realise their full potential in life or to liberate their own personalities. If only dentists realised that they could do more for their patients than the plastic surgeons and the psychiatrists combined! How frequently do we miss the vital clues that patients are embarrassed by their mouths? The smile with the lips kept together; the laugh with the hand in front of the mouth; the head held down whilst in conversation; are all vital clues to the repression of the patients personality caused by their embarrassment over their dental condition. Such signs will be picked up by an aware surgeon within the first few moments of the patient entering the surgery, and he will know that if he is to be really successful in his handling of that patient, then he must treat the whole person and not just the teeth. But how can he do this if he does not know the patient, and how can he know the patient, who is virtually a complete stranger anyway?

The Dentist's Impression

Are the patients really such complete strangers when they enter the surgery? Maybe the dentist is at fault because he has missed many opportunities to gather information. Consider some possibilities. The patient contacts the practice to make an enquiry or make an appointment. Usually this is by telephone, and a trained receptionist may be able to pick up many clues even in a short conversation. Did the patient phone himself, or was it his secretary who made the appointment? That tells you something about the patient. Maybe he (or she) got a friend to phone — that tells you something else. Perhaps he enquired about fees over the phone; which tells you that the money is important to that person for one reason or another. Did he say who recommended him, or again, did he say he was coming for a second opinion, or for a consultation? These are all important things which a dentist who is sensitive and aware will want to know.

He can find out without ever having met the patient, even without the patient having set foot inside the practice if his receptionist is well aware. She can say whether the patient sounded matter of fact or dithery, pleasant or irritable, etc. Of course it is important that the receptionist sounds pleasant herself, and this can be helped tremendously by smiling when she answers the phone. The smile really does come through in the voice!! Remember that the patient is learning about you while you are learning about him, and the way your receptionist deals with him is all part of his knowledge of you. If there is love in your business and among your staff then it will show — and this means that the patient will know instinctively that there is more chance that you will treat him with love. If he has been recommended by another patient he will already have an idea of what you are like and his knowledge of you will be influenced by this second contact.

This patient knowledge will be built up by a third contact, when he actually arrives for his appointment, and he will be influenced firstly by the outside of the premises — is the garden tidy — windows clean — brass shiny, etc. By noticing these things he will realise that you have a standard and self esteem. Then he meets your receptionist — does she answer the door quickly, is she smiling, does she know the patient's name and which dentist the patient is to see, does the patient feel expected and welcomed? And, once inside, are the premises clean and decorated in good taste?

All these points help to create a picture of you in the mind of your patient, help to build up that empathy and mutual understanding which are so essential for a good rapport. Your receptionist now has even more knowledge of your patient; appearance, dress, demeanour, speech, etc. This can be passed on to you. The radiographer may play a part. Maybe the patient has been reading the popular press and is apprehensive of X-rays; — you learned something — and perhaps you will not want to treat a patient who will not allow you to take first class radiographs. It may be better to pass on patients you do not feel compatible with than to find that you have a disgruntled patient because, not having seen the radiographs, your treatment is not so successful as you would have wished.

Finally, the patient is ready to come into the surgery. Your nurse should tell you if he has been calm or agitated in the waiting room, and this will give you another impression of the patient and his personality. The patient will have a better idea of you after seeing your waiting room — is it tasteful decor? What pictures and diplomas or certificates are displayed? All this is part of patient education, of which more later.

Dealing with Patients

I prefer to greet the patients personally as they walk towards the surgery, as I can observe them better this way — the walk, the general standard of health and agility, pallor of skin, brightness of eye and so many other signs, all tell their story. The mannerisms, the bruxing movements and overdeveloped muscles all reveal their standard of occlusal health, and their discomfiture or otherwise with their mouth. In addition, I can 'break the ice' in our relationship more easily by coming to greet the patient. It is ordeal enough going into a strange dental surgery even with all the help which a sympathetic surgeon can show, and this first contact is so important for the surgeon. You never have a second chance to make a good first impression, and whilst one is observing, one can also take the opportunity to show concern and love towards the patient and to establish empathy with him. If you allow the nurse to seat the patient before you 'appear' then you are missing this opportunity and also putting the patient into a mildly stressful situation of being in a strange dental chair, and not knowing what kind of person is going to come in and 'dominate' him. We must understand that the patient is in a 'captive' situation in the dental chair, surrounded by a potentially hurtful environment and is under considerable stress due to the submissive situation in which he finds himself. The sooner you can meet him and assure him that the 'captor' does not pose a further threat the sooner he will be relaxed and reassured.

Consultations should not be carried out with the patient in an easy chair, but in the dental chair, so that he will have overcome that hurdle and be accustomed to the experience. Do not tilt the chair back or even look into the patient's mouth at this stage, because you want the patient to tell you as much as you need to know about himself. And they will tell you virtually anything if you will only allow them to. The temptation to talk at the patient must be resisted and the art of sympathetic listening cultivated. This way you will learn about the person with whom you are dealing. As the wise doctor knows, it is more important to establish what kind of patient has the disease, than to know what kind of disease the patient has.

It is, of course, most important to know if the patient has a specific acute need, and this must be dealt with speedily, painlessly and efficiently. It is no good talking about the future when the patient's needs are painfully and obviously in the present. So that ache must be stopped and that sharp tooth smoothed over before going on. Once having ascertained that the patient's immediate needs have been dealt with, we can carry on.

It is useful at this stage to have a clipboard and make relevant notes so that the patient knows you are paying attention and it is important that you should sit almost directly in front with your eyes at the same level as the patient's, or even lower. (I even kneel down to greet children when they enter the surgery, so that my eyes will be on their level.) On the clipboard you should have a list of potential questions. I say potential questions because most of them may not be asked. — Why? because the questions are not really there to be answered but only to encourage the patient to continue talking. If a lull occurs you can then use questions to start the patient off giving you information about themselves.

Once you know you have the patient relaxed and you have obtained sufficient information for the time being, you can tell the patient something about yourself, and this is the beginning of the patient's education. It is not true that people necessarily know what they want. They may need to be taught their desires and needs, and in this context nobody is going to teach your patients except yourself. More than that, you have to teach the patient to value what you have to offer. People value things according to their knowledge of them, for example a knowledgeable man would put a great value on a Persian carpet, whereas to another it would be just another rug. So you begin by telling the patient that your approach to dentistry is probably different from what he has previously experienced. Immediately the patient knows that there are different types and standards of dentistry and that you aspire to the best. You then go on to explain that to treat him properly you would like to carry out a really thorough four part examination, pre-clinical; clinical; thorough excellent radiographs; and mounted models on an adjustable articulator. As a result of this thorough examination you will then be in a position properly to evaluate his mouth, and to know how the teeth fit in with the way the muscles and bones and joints work. From this you will be able to work out a master plan which will put the whole mouth and jaws into the state best calculated to provide the patient with maximum comfort, appearance and function, and to prolong the life of the teeth for the whole of his life with only basic maintenance. Modern techniques and skills enable us to do this for most people, and save patients from having extensive, expensive, uncomfortable resurrection-type dentistry at a later date.

The treatment can be designed in small units, enabling the patient to have the work done piecemeal if desired. This way the expense need not come in one great blow, and in the meantime the teeth can be put on a 'holding programme' which will maintain the dentition until such time as the proper work can be done. (An amalgam filling may well form part of such a programme.) Of course the patient has nothing to lose except the consultation fee in going ahead with the four part examination and as he has already committed himself to the fee, most will want to go ahead. A patient who does not wish to proceed at this stage is probably not for you and you will make a note to make it easy for them to find another dentist at a convenient moment.

The Clinical Examination

Having completed the pre-clinical examination you are now in a position to go on to the clinical examination. This will start with handing the clipboard visibly to the nurse who sits within sight of the patient whilst the examination is in progress, and visibly makes notes. Put a reassuring hand on the patient's arm and tell them that the chair will move backwards before pressing the button. Ensure the patient is sitting comfortably and then begin with an examination of the muscles of mastication and the temporo mandibular joint. All the time you talk 'through' the patient to the dental nurse. People do not necessarily take notice when they are being talked at, but when they can eavesdrop on a conversation about them, then they are all ears. So you draw the nurse's attention to any irregularities you notice and whilst you are actually talking to the nurse you are really communicating with the patient, and educating him. Don't forget to mention things like overhanging edges on interstitial amalgams, and tell the nurse how this can prejudice the health of the patient's gum. Of course the nurse already knows this, but the patient does not and most will be all agog to know more. And mention that pocket, and the thickened periodontal membrane, the loss of alveolar bone, the tipped teeth, cracked-leaky amalgam and loss of occlusal anatomy. And most important, the aesthetics — if the teeth might look better with a crown etc. And when looking at the X-rays, do not forget to show the patient (through the nurse) what you see. Show the patient how thorough you are by going over every little point. The patient's response to mention of crowns and bridges, or gold fillings, will tell you much, and there is a great deal more you want to know.

Firstly, you may well need to know if the person in the chair is the decision maker. If in a marriage you suspect it is not the patient, for example, then it is pertinent to ask the other spouse to come along to the next appointment. By then you will have the models mounted on an adjustable articulator in terminal hinge position and you will be able to use these and all relevant X-rays to educate both husband and wife. This way you could well end up with two patients instead of one. Alternatively, you could save yourself from the embarrassment of embarking on a course of treatment which, for some reason, did not please the decision-making spouse.

Then you will want to know the patient's attitude towards fees. A simple phrase like 'Is the fee of importance to you?' gives the patient an easy and comfortable opportunity to let you know that money matters to him. In this case, you must make sure he knows he can be kept on a 'holding programme' until such time as he has money available, and that you will not allow his mouth to deteriorate until he can afford to go ahead with the 'master plan'. And remind him that the master plan has been designed to be carried out in easy stages. If he wants to know about fees, then you must tell him.

Fees and Patients

How do you set your fee? Well, you must charge an appropriate fee, i.e. a fee which will allow you to do your best work using the best technicians and the best materials, and give you a fair reward for the time and knowledge expended, and which can be explained reasonably to the patient.

In order to put things in perspective, it is useful to know that Reiner carried out a 'survey of surveys' into the reasons why patients decide to go to a particular dentist. Fees came fifth, at the bottom of the list, after (1) Personality of the dentist, (2) Reputation of the dentist, (3) Quality of workmanship, (4) Convenience (eg. location, parking, ease of obtaining appointments).

Let us talk a little more about fees. You must have a proper set fee for your work. This is your fee. Not your usual fee, but your fee. This fee will not necessarily be invariable. It can vary according to the type of patient you are dealing with. Here it is pertinent to divide your patients into four groups, 1, 2, 3 and 4. Groups one and two are the informed patients who have come to you because they want fine dentistry. Groups three and four are your uninformed patients. Group four are those who do not know and do not want to know about good dentistry. There are plenty of dentists around who are only too happy to cater for these people by providing basic dentistry, and you should have no qualms about making it easy for these patients to find a dentist who will cater for their needs. He will think you are a super chap for referring patients to him, and one day he is going to get a patient in his surgery who does want extensive restoration work which is beyond him. He may send that patient to you, and that patient will be worth ten times more than the dozen patients you may have sent his way. So do make it easy for patients who do not fit in with your style of practice to go elsewhere, and do not be bothered about it in your conscience.

Type three patients are those who are uneducated about good dentistry, but who are able and potentially willing to learn, and who could afford to pay the fee if they knew the true value of what they were getting. These patients can be anything from an office girl to a millionaire. Many wealthy and important people find great difficulty in having their mouths maintained to the standards they would apply to their houses, gardens or their cars. They would welcome the chance to learn, and to have first class treatment. At the other end of the scale many an office worker would jump at the chance to buy good dentistry if she was taught the value of it. People buy what they value and are prepared to save up and make sacrifices for what they want. They afford holidays in the Caribbean or Mediterranean, expensive hi-fi equipment, hair-dos and beauty treatments, vast wardrobes of clothes etc. and they bother to save up to buy these things because they have been educated to value them and because they are high on their list of priorities. It is up to you to educate your patients so that fine dentistry is esteemed and high in their scale of values. A good holiday may be enjoyable but it does not last. Good dentistry does.

If these class three patients can be educated to value good dentistry they can advance to a higher class. Most of your new patients, particularly in the early days of your practice will start off as class threes and will form the backbone of the practice. If you educate them they may end up as class ones or class twos.

Class one and class two patients are those who are educated about good dentistry and value it. The class one patient is not only well educated but is also well able to pay the fee. And the fee he pays is your fee, which we have already discussed. He pays with gratitude because he knows he is getting value for money. These people show their gratitude in a variety of ways: by their warmth towards the dentist, treating him as a trusted friend; by their loyalty and regular return visits; by verbal thanks or grateful letters; by gifts which can be small or large; by prompt settlement of the account; by referring their friends, and in many other little ways. These things are the dentist's joy in the knowledge of a job well done and appreciated. They make life worthwhile, and the ill feeling caused by bad debts is avoided. Ultimately it all stems from the love arm in that cross of life. There are actions and reactions, and if you act with love in providing your patients with a valued service, then they can only react with love towards you in appreciation.

Class two patients are also well educated and value good dentistry, but for one reason or another they find themselves genuinely unable to afford it. If their poverty is temporary, eg they are going through 'a bad patch', the solution is to maintain their mouths and keep them on a holding programme until such time as their temporary poverty is past and they can become a class one patient again. The fees for these patients may justifiably and charitably be lowered. But they must understand what you have done, and that you are giving them a reduction in fee for the moment. This is important not only for the promotion of good will but also when the 'poor period' is past, it makes it easy to revert to 'the fee' again. Such arrangements might also be made for those whose poverty is more permanent — but obviously such cases should be rare (possibly the patient of many years standing) and should be carefully considered.

Patient Motivation

Having classified your patient in the above groups there is yet something else you will want to know, and that is the patient's basic motivation. I have seen the basic types of motivation classified as the 4 R's. Reward, Romance, Recognition and Resurrection. Reward, of course, is our old friend financial gain, and Resurrection is often written down as personal survival or self preservation. We all possess all of these motivations together but in varying degrees. In each individual, one will probably be more dominant than the others. It is most important that you do not offer gold restorations to an attractive young lady with a Romance dominant personality. She will much prefer porcelain crowns on her back teeth and will shy away from gold. On the other hand, someone whose dominant motivation is self preservation (the Resurrection type) will go for gold every time, even at the expense of appearance, because it is stronger, better wearing and longer lived. Reward dominant people can have peculiar ideas — from Scrooge-like determination not to part with their money (they often will pay for themselves but want something cheap for the family) to a desire for it to be known and obvious what they have spent their money on. The ultimate in this last was a husband who insisted on his wife's beautiful natural looking crowns being replaced with nice obvious white ones so that people would know he had paid to have it done! Of course, recognition played a part in this also. Patients thus motivated want it to be recognised that in their wisdom they have chosen the best dentist (remember those certificates on the waiting-room wall).

Another question you will want answered is why the patient has not had good regular dentistry before. The three most common causes cited are 'it hurts', 'I can't afford it' and 'I don't have the time'. It is important to know these things so that patients can learn that with local anaesthetics, relative analgesia, hypnosis, intravenous sedation and other things, we have means of ensuring that dentistry is painless if not actually enjoyable. One will take even greater care than usual over these patients to minimise their fears, and phrase comments to build up their confidence. Cost has already been dealt with, but patients must be educated to value good dentistry and raise it up in their order of priorities. Of course, most can afford it if they want to. And the same goes for time. If people value something enough they will find the time for it. How many hours are spent watching television — playing golf or cards — watching sport etc? It is all a question of education and priorities and such "reasons" for not having good dentistry are really invalid excuses.

But there is a fourth reason why people don't have good dentistry and it is probably the most difficult one of all to handle. It is when a patient thinks they have already been having good dentistry. This is a delicate situation, because the previous dentist might be an old and trusted friend who did his best. You might think it a pity he didn't know any better but you don't tell the patient this. Use your radiographs and models to show him what needs doing and let him draw his own conclusions. If the patient remarks that you are more thorough than Mr. X, or why didn't Mr. X advise this, then you can gently point out that there has been an explosion of new knowledge and techniques in dentistry and that you have made a big effort to keep up with this.

You will also want to know about your patients' personality, and their confidence level. Are they embarrassed by their dentition? Does this affect their personality? It must do. Be on the look out for that rotated or instanding tooth, or that unpleasant stain or mark. Ask if it worries him or her. Listen carefully for the guarded reply. It doesn't matter what the patient's mother thinks or what their friends think. It doesn't even matter what you think. It's what the patient thinks that matters and if a woman thinks she is ugly, then she is, and she will lack confidence because of it. Remove the cause of the ugliness and the confidence returns, frequently with dramatic results. Shy, retiring young girls return six months later for a check up as confident women, who have gained promotion in their work. Instead of looking shyly towards the ground as they creep into your surgery, they walk briskly in, hand outstretched, smile on the face and confidence simply oozing from them. Their personality is liberated. You have done more than any psychiatrist. And this is not confined to the fair sex, men are just as concerned, and just as inhibited by a poor smile. Improve the smile and you improve the person. The smile is such a basic gesture, a really deep primitive social necessity. Success in our business life, our love life and our social life all depend on it. And the more confident it is, the more compelling the personality behind it. But it is not only the smile which affects confidence — comfort and function affect this too. You cannot give of your best at a business luncheon if it hurts to eat and you are in pain all the while. An inability to masticate the food either results in indigestion (helped on by the stress of the need for a successful outcome of the talking) or in food left on the plate. This can be interpreted either as a lack of appreciation of what is provided by the host, nervousness, lack of confidence, or just plain lack of interest. So it is immensely important to find out all these things about your patients.

Add all these things together, and join them with the knowledge you have gained from your occlusal examination (the presence of facial pain, headaches, nausea, sleepless nights, which may well be due to dental causes, which are not only debilative but will also depress the patient's personality) and you will see for yourself that you can do more for your patient than almost any other specialist. Truly, dentistry is in no way the Cinderella of the medical sciences. We have a tremendously important contribution to make and we should be excited at the opportunities open to us, and very aware of the responsibility which lies in our hand.

❧ 4 ❧

Know Your Work

Know your work? Of course you do, you are a fully qualified dentist with several years' experience in practice, and you were a student at the best dental school. But your school was concerned to teach you the basics of your profession, so perhaps there just might be more to learn if only you knew where to find it. And have those several years in practice blunted the edge of your perception, made you feel a little smug and even self-satisfied? It can easily happen to all of us.

Of course there is more to learn. Knowledge never stops advancing, and tremendous advances in understanding have been made in the dental profession since the middle of our century. And these advances are making tremendous changes in the way dentistry is being practised, changes which are occurring with great rapidity right under our noses. We live in a time of rapid change. Speedy communication of ideas means that changes in theory and practice that would have taken a generation in previous centuries now take place in a few years, and changes which previously might have taken a lifetime are now accomplished in little more than a decade. So we must be adaptable if we are to keep up.

Three Tiers of Dentistry

In the developed countries of the world the trend is for dentistry to be carried out at different levels. The basic level, or 'tier one dentistry', (fig.11) is mainly concerned with quantity, and is provided for people whose financial commitment is subsidised one way or another. In Britain, this is done through the National Health Service, in Europe and in the U.S.A. through various insurance schemes. Such dentistry is mainly tooth orientated, and is concerned principally with the repair of damage caused by dental disease. This is the basic dentistry as taught in the dental schools of the world.

Many dentists have become disillusioned with the restrictions, and lack of fulfilment and work satisfaction which goes with the quantity orientated style, and have moved on to a second type of practice. This seeks to place more emphasis on quality, and is fee orientated. The patient is required to pay the full fee for the work, and the dentist undertakes to use more loving care and attention in carrying out his procedures. This 'tier two' type of dentistry is basically not very different to that done by Tier one dentists, but is carried out to a higher standard both of work and service. In Britain this is known as 'going private'. In the U.S.A. it is giving rise to all sorts of innovations even to franchise dentistry, where the surgeon joins a group and the group advertise collectively across the country. Frequently, surgeons try to combine tiers one and two, especially when they are in the process of changing over from one to the other, but ideally Tier two dentistry needs a wholehearted commitment, because if some of the patients are Tier one, then a Tier one attitude tends to pervade the staff and the set-up of the practice. This 'tier one attitude' will mitigate against 'tier two' patients who will feel they are not getting the service to make the extra fee worthwhile. So the changeover is as much concerned with attitude of mind as with knowledge or higher standards of work.

Over and above these two tiers, is emerging a new type of practice, 'tier three' dentistry. This is not simply concerned with teeth or even the mouth, but sees the patient as a human being, and tries to treat the whole person. It realises that good dentistry can be free of pain and stress and can combine with first class aesthetics to give the patient health and confidence. It can liberate the patient's personality with tremendous effect in their social life, business life and love life. Such dentistry is concerned with health, rather than treatment of disease, and it seeks to understand the whole environment into which the dental work is being placed, so that the patient can maintain his natural dentition for life with the best possible results in appearance, function, comfort and confidence. Tier three dentistry is sometimes called 'holistic' dentistry, and it will be readily appreciated that the most important thing for the aspiring holistic dentist to achieve is the right attitude of mind towards the patient, and towards himself. We are where we think we are, and our own self image is so important, as was discussed in Chapter two. Our attitude towards the patient must also be very carefully fostered because the holistic dentist is concerned with people, and he will want the whole of his practice to reflect his attitude of mind.

In terms of his work, such a dentist will mainly be interested in two things, understanding of function, and excellence. It is most important to differentiate between excellence and perfection. Perfection is unattainable. The more we know about perfection, the more we appreciate that we have not achieved it. Artists in any field, or even saints and holy people have the same problem. The great ballet dancers know that they have never given a perfect performance, and great painters know that they have never painted a perfect picture. Saints also realise their own imperfections and rely on the forgiveness of God for their lapses. An understanding of this is so important if one is to avoid being plagued by scruples, and it must be realised that if one has done one's best, then this is sufficient. Excellence is the best that one can achieve at any given moment, whilst realising that there are always higher standards which can be reached. The best that can be achieved in any given set of circumstances may be limited by various factors, the knowledge of the surgeon, the conditions under which he is trying to work, the co-operation of the patient and training of staff, the availability of materials etc. Most of these can be improved one way or another. The surgeon can improve his knowledge, and he can improve the conditions under which he works by updating equipment, redesigning accommodation, etc. Staff can be trained and encouraged to do better, and a stock of potentially useful materials can be maintained.

Patients

Patients may present problems. They may, for example, be 'difficult', or have irritating habits. Many of these irritations can be helped in two ways. Firstly, the surgeon can improve his personal approach and skill in relaxing the patient. The best analgesic in the world is a good chairside manner, and an understanding attitude of mind. It is important to do everything one can to put the patient at ease and inspire confidence. This starts with the attitude of the staff, and is reinforced by the decor and colour scheme of the premises. No harsh or exciting colours should be used, only those colours which are known to be psychologically relaxing. And the surgeon should do everything confidently and purposefully. No sudden movements such as putting the chair back without telling the patient, no bright lights in the eyes or harsh sudden noise, but always a reassuring touch of the hand. And the touch when working in the mouth should be firm enough to inspire confidence, but not rough or harsh. This is most important. The over-gentle touch does not inspire confidence, but smacks of an unsure and incapable approach. The rough, harsh touch lacks love and smacks of lack of concern for the patient, and encourages an unfavourable reaction.

But even when all these things are done well there will still be patients who are difficult because of their nature or their past history. It is very difficult for someone who has had a bad experience to regain his confidence and every help should be provided in the form of various analgesics. We have such a wide range available nowadays — local anaesthetics, relative analgesia, intravenous sedation, hypnotism and sophrology, full general anaesthesia, and even acupuncture. Surely one or another, or even a combination of these, can be found to suit any individual, and enable the surgeon to achieve excellence.

Finally, there are those patients whose personality clashes with the surgeons. In most of these cases, the patient will make it easy by finding another dentist, but if this doesn't happen, and it becomes obvious that things will not improve, then the surgeon should make it easy for the patient to go somewhere else. Frequently the mere suggestion that the dentist thinks he and the patient are incompatible will cause the patient to change radically, and become a reformed character, because he has come to respect the standard of excellence offered, and hadn't realised just how difficult he was being. Remember that we cannot like everyone, and we are not expected to. There is a difference in liking people and loving people. We can even love our enemies, but this does not mean we want to live in their own back yard. To love someone is to wish them well and hope good things for them, to be concerned for their welfare. You can do all this without necessarily liking them, although it is more difficult than loving someone you like. But that is the challenge, and it is so much more rewarding in so many ways to come to like people through love. The greatest gift is to understand other people's minds. The person who can truly put himself in another's place and understand his point of view has a tremendous advantage in life, and especially in dentistry. This is called empathy.

Over and above all, the tier three dentist will not just be interested in the patient's teeth, but will see the teeth as simply the cutting edge of a machine which consists of muscles and bones, joints, nerves and ligaments. He will want to be knowledgeable on the ways to set the chewing machine into a harmonious method of working which will provide maximum comfort and minimum stress. And he will be well aware of the penalties for failure in an unhappy patient.

The symptoms of 'occlusal disease' which result from disharmony in the chewing machine can be very far-reaching, and are often so far removed from the teeth that the patient does not associate them with dentistry at all, and seeks help from other members of the healing professions, doctors, physiotherapists, osteopaths, acu-puncturists, etc. The symptoms can be described by various name-tags — migraine, neuralgia, sinusitis, ear-ache, neck and shoulder pain, and chronic headache. These are but some of the different words that are frequently used by patients to describe their aches and pains. Why are the sites and type of pain so varied? The answer is that, with any machine under stress, the part which gives way is always the weakest link in the chain, and since all humans are different, in each person the breakdown will occur in the weakest part in his particular body. It can be either the teeth which fracture under pressure, or the supporting tissues which break down, or it can be the joints, or the neuro-musculature. But how do the teeth contribute to this state of affairs? And why are all these muscles so important? Surely the body has been designed to cope with the functions it is required to perform? Or could it be that the body can become overstressed by being made to work at times and in ways which are not associated with normal function? It is so important for dentists to find the answers to these questions.

The elimination of stress must be our major objective. Any dentistry done in a stress-free mouth must be more successful, and a stress-free mouth must be much more comfortable. The function is bound to be better because it is more harmonious and it is a fact that good function usually goes along with good appearance and harmonious aesthetics.

This is an exposition of philosophy and understanding. It is not intended to be a textbook of the how and the why; these things have already been more than adequately covered in the excellent books by Peter Dawson[1] and Nathan Alan Shore[3] and I heartily recommend these books to the aspiring dentist. In reading these books, practitioners will also find more than adequate guidance in the search for excellence with regard to cavity preparations and impression taking, and also in case planning.

As a final word on the subject of 'know your work', it is worth reiterating that the absolute key to success is to start with good full mouth radiographs, and models mounted on an anatomical articulator. And it is so necessary to keep going to courses and seminars to continue the learning process, and to meet other like-minded dentists who can reinforce and sustain each others' momentum and thinking. It is difficult to aspire to do the best, and understanding of the principles involved is not easy. It helps to listen to different lecturers, saying the same thing in different ways, and listening to the same lecturer repeatedly, until finally one really hears what is being said. At this point one can say that one really owns the knowledge, because one understands it.

The pursuit of excellence is a never ending journey. There is always some new depth of understanding to be plumbed. This is what makes dentistry an enriching and challenging profession, because the fascination of new knowledge and deeper understanding is a lifetime vocation, and a continuing joy.

✦ 5 ✦

Apply Your Knowledge

The most worthwhile investment for any dentist is in his own knowledge. Any money spent on improving one's own knowledge must bear a percentage reward which far outweighs any other investment.

But, in order to bear fruit, knowledge must be applied. It is no good going on courses and then returning home to one's practice and forgetting all about it. Alas! This last is all too frequently the sequel to most postgraduate education.

Why Knowledge Should be Applied

The reason why knowledge should be applied is usually because the routine in the practice goes on in the same old way; the same number of patients are booked in, the same attitude pervades the staff, and the energy and determination needed to change the way things have been going on is squeezed out by the pressures of everyday dentistry. Then a week goes by and the determination is much less. Another week, and the postgraduate course is nothing but a memory.

It is therefore necessary, having completed a course, to make a firm commitment to do certain things immediately on one's return. This must be set down in writing before one reaches the practice on Monday morning or it will be lost. One dentist I know writes these things on a notepad whilst sitting in the aeroplane on the way home. He covers which things he wants to change in the way the practice is run and what he needs to order in the way of equipment. He hands the list of equipment to his secretary, and knows that when the things arrive that will be an added incentive to use them in order to recoup the outlay in money. And he personally will have no excuse not to use new techniques 'because he hasn't got the right tools in the practice'. This is the easy part.

The difficult part is in doing what needs to be done to change patterns of work by the staff, and this needs motivation. Your own enthusiasm is usually the best motivator in the world, but one must be careful to carry the staff along in a positive way. If they are left feeling that they have been doing it all wrong all these years, they can easily become disgruntled and hostile towards the proposed changes. So make sure they feel encouraged in a positive way, that they feel they are involved in something exciting which will make better use of their particular talents. And make sure they know their talents are appreciated. They can also be helped to realise that by doing things better they personally will grow spiritually and become more fulfilled. As Abraham Maslow[2] points out, the best businesses are those where the employees are involved to some extent in the why and wherefore of decision making, and feel part of the organisation to the point where they can grow and become self actualising. In this way love can pervade the whole staff of the organisation and productivity and profitability improve. But the opposite can happen and a member of the staff find that they do not like the new methods. In this case, they can become resentful and obstructive. If no way can be found around this, then it may be necessary to help that person find employment in another practice more congenial to their ideas. It can be done in a loving and friendly attitude of mind. I know of one young dentist who had bought his practice only a year or so before and the old staff were so imbued in the ways of his predecessor that they refused to change. He had to get rid of all three of them and start anew. Fortunately, he had a choice of applicants and was able to employ one of the many consultancy firms that are around nowadays, to help him find the girls whose temperament and psychological make up were in harmony with himself and with what he wanted to achieve. His attitude can be very helpful to many of us. There are so many advisory bodies around for all aspects of business management, and there is no need to put up with square pegs in round holes.

Carrying one's staff along with one is important, and will make the next part of change so much easier. That is, of course, changing one's premises. In order to accommodate some new ideas, the physical set up of the practice may have to be changed and this may involve moving staff around so that they work in different rooms, or even moving walls or building partitions in order to introduce some new concept, or even moving premises altogether. So many opportunities here for the unwary boss to get on the wrong side of the staff. So many opportunities for the thinking dentist to involve his staff and utilise their ideas, so that in the end they will almost feel that they have done it all themselves. How nice when they think 'we enlarged the laboratory' rather than 'the boss did it — can't think why'.

Of course, these things need a great deal of thought and time, and it cannot be done whilst rushing around seeing patients. It is essential to 'cross off time' just to sit, and think, and look, and talk to people. Usually half a day would barely be enough, and a whole day crossed off is better. It is important to tell the staff to ensure that one is not bothered by day to day work. The dentist is out if patients call or 'phone, and ordinary mail must temporarily be set aside. If you are behindhand and need a day to catch up on your routine, then take one, but keep it as a separate day from your forward planning day.

Forward Planning

Once you are into your forward planning day and you have time to think, then there are other things you can ponder. First, the appointment book. Do you want to go on working the same routine? If not, what are you going to do about it? Do you want to apply your specialised knowledge, in which case how much time are you going deliberately to set aside for it? And if you set time aside for bridge preparations, then you must also set aside time to fit them. One person I know colour codes his appointment book. He can only take on two new patients a week. He knows this, and also knows the time when he can expect them. His book does not get into a muddle and he ends up doing the sort of work he wants to do because he has designed things that way. But he has also designed so much more because he has taken time out to think about things and work things out. In short, he has a plan.

One should use the time on the regular planning days to set goals and plan how to achieve them. Goals can be short and long term. The divisions of the calendar give various opportunities for review of situations, weekly, monthly, quarterly and yearly, two yearly, five yearly, ten yearly etc. The weekly and monthly reviews can be fairly short. The quarterly should be longer, and the yearly longer still. All should be carefully thought out. Years pass by surprisingly quickly, and if we are not careful ten years go by with very little having been achieved. One looks at others who have got on with life and wonders 'how did he get there, and I'm still here?' The answer is that he planned it out.

What sort of dentist do you want to be in ten years' time? What sort of person do you want to be? What sort of house would you really like to live in? What do you want for your family in terms of education, travel, etc? What do you want to own, to see? What talents do you want to develop, and what skills to improve upon? What achievements do you aspire to? All these things will have a bearing on your practice, because you will need both time and money to accomplish them. Thus the most important considerations are how much time you wish to spend at work and how much money you need to finance yourself in fulfilling your aspirations.

Take a piece of paper and write all these things down. Then plan how you are going to achieve them, and this means applying your knowedge more profitably, and increasing your knowledge to the point where you will attract the sort of patient who can help you achieve your goal. This will mean a steady upgrading of everything in the practice, better equipment, nicer furnishing and decoration and better and more loving attitudes from staff to patients. Plan all this into your goal, so that gradually, over a period of time, all is achieved, major expenses being paid for by major breakthroughs in application of knowledge. And this is important in avoiding unnecessary stress.

Stress and Competence

Stress is not necessarily a bad thing. We are told it is a killer and so it can be. But it is also a part of life. Enjoyment is stress; watching a football match or even falling in love is extremely stressful, so stress is part of life. It has been said that to be completely stress free one would have to be dead! But obviously stress can be excessive and then it can be extremely harmful to health. This needs to be said because introducing new ideas and techniques is stressful. And trying to achieve unrealistic goals can be extremely and unnecessary dangerous. So make your goals high enough to give you something to aspire to but not so high as to be impossible. And remember that 'the best-laid schemes o' mice an' men Gang aft agley' and if circumstances look like preventing you from achieving your goal, then be adaptable enough to change your plans and modify your goals.

Do not be afraid of stress particularly in applying new knowledge and techniques. Loren Miller has a wonderful phrase, 'one's comfort zone'. This is the place where we are working comfortably, under minimal stress. The comfort zone is the product of our competence and our confidence. Some people have a very good idea of their own competence, and their confidence and competence coincide. They are comfortable doing work which they know they are competent to do. And there they stay, never achieving anything more demanding, but doing what they know extremely well. But the majority of dentists have confidence levels way below their own competence. They seldom try to achieve their own capability because they lack self confidence and do not feel comfortable working to their limits.

If you would improve then you not only have to work right up to your capability, but you have to learn new techniques. New techniques have to be tried for the first time, and this involves most of us going out of our comfort zone because we are not sure how we will fare, and fear we are beyond our level of competence. So improving one's techniques involves entering a stressful area, putting ourselves to the test by applying new knowledge. We should not let this worry us unduly. The basic ground rules and basic understanding are there and if we stick to our well known principles we will not go far wrong. And don't be put off if it doesn't all work out perfectly the first time. The patient is still better off than if you had not had the courage to put yourself to the test. And after a few successful attempts, it is wonderful to feel how one's competence level has been raised to the point where one feels comfortable with the new technique. This in turn stimulates one's confidence and one is happier to go out and learn more advanced techniques, confident that with careful thought and application one can also put them into operation successfully.

Two other things are necessary to know in applying one's knowledge. Never forget that everyone is unique. Firstly, because you are unique your practice will be unique: it will reflect your personality. And the type of work done and the type of patient who attends will reflect your application of your knowledge. Secondly the standard of dental education of your patients is unique. Being unique only you can educate your patients to admire and aspire to the type of dentistry which you practice. If you aspire to the best dentistry then you will attract the best patients and they will go out and talk about you, like missionaries for good dentistry. And remembering that like recommends like, you will gradually be building up a practice of really first class patients. Most new patients who come into your surgery will expect the best before they even arrive. There is no competition at the top because there are not enough dentists to carry out all the really good dentistry needed if people only realise it is available.

Know your work, and apply your knowledge. But in order to apply your knowledge, you will have to carry your patients along with you. It is pointless to take your harp to a party if no-one will ask you to play!

It is very important that one's patients want to have the sort of work that the dentist can do. This will only happen if they are convinced of the need for it, and have absolute confidence in the dentist. This in turn demands three things from the dentist; absolute honesty, loving the patient enough to want to do your best for them, and an ability to communicate with them. Honesty and love are better than all the sales gimmicks in the world. And the four part examination using pre-clinical and clinical examinations, full mouth X-rays and study models mounted on an anatomical articulator, is the finest means of educating the patient. Once the patient can see the problem he can accept the answer. Even if it takes several years to complete the master plan, he will be prepared to persevere. It is surprising how many dentists spend most of the time talking to patients about proposed treatment instead of explaining the problem. If they did so they would find that their treatment plan would follow on logically. Patients would accept it easily and with the minimum of discussion. They can also appreciate that the dentist has taken account of their own personal needs, their temperament, station in life, ability to pay, the needs of their business, social and love life. He will also be aware that the dentist has taken trouble to find out how to achieve the desired goal in the most economical and effective way. Remember that sins are of two basic kinds, positive and negative. We can sin positively by doing something, by making a mistake. Negative sins can be just as damaging if not more so. To leave undone that which one ought to have done is just as bad as to do what one ought not to have done. Patients quickly sense whether the dentist is applying himself and doing his best. They enjoy the fact that the dentist is taking extra trouble, using a magnifying loup for example to ensure a high standard. And how rewarding it all is for the dentist. As Michaelangelo said, 'trifles make perfection, and perfection is no trifle'. There is no pleasure in doing slipshod work, no lift for the soul, no sense of achievement. But the rewards of doing one's best are beyond all expectations. A patient recently told me that it had taken her four weeks to appreciate the immensity of the achievement of the dentistry she had received. The more she thought about it the more she appreciated it. She smiled a lot, became radiant, held her head higher and generally appeared confident, poised and assured – and all because of good dentistry. She had already talked her girl friend into having the same kind of dentistry. What spiritual joy for the dentist to have his work talked about in such phrases, what uplift for the soul, what encouragement to continue the search for excellence, to continue the 'immensity of achievement'! All this can be yours.

Know yourself, know your patient, know your work and apply your knowledge. You will not only help your patients but you will find your own soul too.

✝6✝

Love

The Greeks had three words for love: *eros* — or erotic love, *philos*, or intellectual love, and *agape*, that selfless love of the souls of others, which is characterised by the christian word charity. Throughout this chapter the word love will be used in its charitable connotation.

Love is the most important thing in the world. With love, all that is finest in human life comes to its fruition; without love, vileness and bestiality abound and life becomes a living hell. Philosophers and religions throughout the centuries have testified to the importance of love.

Unfortunately, the appreciation of love was undermined by Freud, who considered it unimportant, if not irrelevent. The problem was that Freud based his observations on his experience with diseased minds, and therefore his conclusions were out of balance, rather like a doctor who sees the whole of human life in terms of diseased bodies without ever relating his ideas to healthy people. It is important to study physiology before one studies pathology. Freud was followed by the so-called behaviourist school of psychology, who extended Darwinism to include the idea that, since man descended from animals then his behavioural patterns would be similar to those of animals. Thus the working of the human mind could be related to the way animals behave. This is obviously a very limited approach.

Later people like William James began to question this thesis. They realised that there was much more to man than appeared to most psychologists, and that most people were not even beginning to achieve their full potential. From this emerged what is now called third force psychology, the best known proponant of which is Dr. Abraham Maslow.[2]

Maslow decided to study healthy human minds, to learn something about mental physiology. He thought that if he could find out what happened when men achieved something approaching their full potential, then he could see what was different about people who did not. By studying health he could see why the unhealthy state had developed. Maslow found that healthy people had achieved their own capability, that their personality had in fact become an actuality. So he called them 'self-actualising' people. He tried to determine the most healthy people in the world and studied their personalities by every means at his disposal. A remarkable pattern emerged from which he was able to identify the factors leading to mental health and 'self-actualisation'.

Man's unconscious mind or 'id', he discovered, was not just bad, evil, or dangerous, and always having to be suppressed by his higher consciousness, as Freud had postulated, but in the healthy 'self-actualising' individual, the subconscious was loving, positive and creative. He also discovered that one of the most important needs of mankind is love; if we are to be healthy, then we must love and be loved. Many psychopathologists now consider the thwarting of the needs of love as a prime cause of mental disease. Love hunger (according to Maslow) is a deficiency disease like avitaminosis. To be truly healthy we must seek to understand more about love and try to live our lives in a loving atmosphere. This in turn will encourage other people to love. But to love involves the difficult process of dropping our defences and overcoming our own fears. Love is giving as well as receiving, and we must all try to learn to teach it, to initiate it, and even to predict it, or the world is lost to hostility and suspicion. With love, people can become themselves, and go on to fulfil their own uniqueness.

Love and the Family

The first place in which we should appreciate love is in our family. One cannot do anything about one's own child-hood, because that is past, but one can determine to do something as a husband or wife, and as a parent, to create a loving atmosphere in one's own home. The home is the most important place for most of us in life. It is that place from which we launch into the world, and to which we return after the toil of the day. It should be a haven of love from which we can emerge refreshed; a well of love from which we can draw living water to take with us into the world to sustain ourselves and others. Truly, the home is the basis for all things in life and if we are unhappy and insecure at home, then it is almost impossible to succeed outside. Why? Because if we come from an atmosphere of contention then we are going to carry that with us into our day. And how can we enjoy our day if we know we have to return to an unwelcoming environment at night? Our irritability will transmit itself to those around us, be they staff or patients, and our business will not be as happy or run as well as it might.

The place to start building up one's love is therefore at home, and there is a right order of priorities. First comes one's marriage partner. Remember, when you marry you leave mother and father and cleave unto your spouse. Parents immediately take second place. The first question to ask yourself, therefore, is 'am I being a good husband (wife)'? This is the prime relationship and it should be worked at as such. It is possible to have a good marriage just as it is possible to have a good practice. The requirements are similar, much love, much hard work and understanding, and a sense of determined commitment as one works towards one's goal. People are apt to think of others who are successful as 'lucky'. It doesn't seem to matter if one has a good business or a good marriage, or even a beautiful home, people will say it is luck. Of course, one may have taken one's opportunities, but basically achievements all require hard work and dedication. Most people who fail do so because they let things slip through their fingers; because they don't have enough self-discipline. The result is that their opportunities come to nothing, because the fruits are dissipated on the worthless tinsel of life. Many things give a moment of pleasure, which is soon past; and then the cost has to be counted.

Adultery is a good example. It involves spending one's time, energies and money outside the family, which means that the family and home suffer to that extent. For oneself, there is the mental problem associated with the act. People investigating longevity consider that adulterers can subtract a few years off their life expectancy because of the stress associated with the act. And that is presumed to be pleasure! How much better to make one's effort towards the worthwhile things which bring deep contentment and lasting joy. The most worthwhile thing in life is a good marriage, so work at yours and constantly be striving to raise your standard of excellence just as you do in regard to your dentistry. Are you a good marriage partner? Well, are you?

Now ask yourself how you can improve, and make a symbolic gesture to make sure you do something about it. Overcome your fear and anxiety and start to make those acts of love. Love begets love. It encourages people to love in return. Love is patient, it bears with the other person's fears and anxieties until they feel they can drop their defences and reciprocate. Love hopes for all things. Love is truth. Love is kind and does not envy. Love is not puffed up, and does not flaunt itself. Love endures and grows upon itself, especially in marriage, where the parties can build love upon love until they achieve a veritable monument.

From the love of the husband and wife come the children. Flesh of one's flesh and blood of one's body. They are the second most important people in life after your spouse, and the second most worthy of your love. Your love can help your children to healthy psychological growth so that they can be a joy to you at home and a force for good in the world. Children need a secure, warm friendly and loving atmosphere with kindly discipline in which to grow. Ashley Montague, the anthropologist, says, 'There is now good evidence which leads us to believe that not only does a baby want to be loved, but that it wants to love and that all of its drives are oriented in the direction of receiving and giving love'; furthermore, he pointed out that deprivation of love means that the child could find it very difficult to give it even as an adult. Dr. Henry Chapin and many others have pointed to cases where children actually died from lack of love, although their other basic needs were well cared for. Frustration of the love-need leads to psychopathology. Satisfaction leads to healthy individuals and there is nothing more rewarding in this world for parents than healthy, happy children who are growing and achieving to the best of their ability.

Ask yourself the question 'Am I a good parent?' Do you provide your family with a sufficiency of love? Do they really know the feeling of belonging? How can you improve things?

The third set of people in your hierarchy of love are your parents. Are you a good son or daughter? This extension of your family to cover the past generation can be very rewarding for yourself and for your children. And if you do not love your parents, what example are you showing? It can be very difficult, as parents are often awkward people; sometimes they have lacked love and wronged their children. One must try to forgive these things, even if it is difficult to forget. Sometimes it may be better to love one's parents from a distance rather than fight with them at close quarters. Always remember that marriages come first and that parents should not interfere or undermine their child's marriage in any way. Most parents do love their children, even if some find difficulty in showing it. So, are you a good son or daughter; and what are you going to do about improving that?

Love and the Practice

Once you have built up your love at home you can carry it with you out into the world and the first place will be your practice. Here you will be able to influence two sets of people — your staff and your patients.

The first people to benefit from your loving attitude will be your staff. Your example will beget a loving attitude in them which will be reflected in the whole of your practice, and will be most obvious to people outside. Staff will not only have a love and respect for you, but they will learn to love each other and build up an attitude of understanding and co-operation throughout the whole of your practice. People will learn to stand in for each other and to support each other. And your consideration for them and their welfare will encourage them to grow in consideration for you and your well-being. By being loving and by setting high standards of consideration and service, you beget these things in others. And since they support you in all things, you will find it much easier to support them in their needs; be understanding when they are sick, or have other problems; be solicitous for their wellbeing if ever they have to leave your employment, or when they retire. Try to make provision for benefits, insurances, pensions and related matters. Find them help with their taxes, so that they pay the minimum legally required of them.

In return, the staff will love the patients on your behalf. The patients are the most important people in the practice, for without them no one would earn any money. Loving the patients will ensure that they receive the finest treatment from you, and the finest and most considerate service from your staff. Nothing is as disarming as love. Even difficult patients succumb, as the demons of the underworld succumbed to Orpheus and his lute. The smile in the voice on the telephone, the attitude that nothing is too much trouble, make it very hard for the 'difficult' patient to take advantage because it becomes clear to them that it is they who are being difficult. But knowing your patients may lead you to grade them into psychological types and try to deal with them differently. Quite frankly, my experience has been that typecasting a patient can be a recipe for disaster — Give a dog a bad name . . . It encourages staff to take up attitudes in order to deal with the type of person who is expected. This shows, and the patients resent it; love also shows and the patients respond, they respond with love, and stop being difficult.

They become the best person of their type instead of the worst. There are actions and reactions; and if the dentist and the staff act in a loving way then it becomes extremely difficult for the patients to react in any other way than with love. Then practice becomes a true joy because patients co-operate and understand when, for example, they cannot have the appointment they want, or if for technical reasons they cannot have their prosthesis just at the time they would have liked. They also understand when (as happens in every establishment from time to time) things go wrong. Who has not had the experience of the patient coming for an appointment at the wrong time? Or of technical work which was inadequate and could not be fitted? Or, indeed, of times when the patient arrived on time but the prosthesis didn't!! Love and absolute honesty, these are the surest things to have on one's side in times like these.

Finally, love for the patient will involve treating the whole person. This is not just suiting the work to the patient's needs and personality, it is understanding that we live in time, and that patients change. We are all different people from what we were a year ago or even a day ago, because events take place which change our appreciation of things, our outlook, and even our reactions and the way we feel. Love will try and understand when the patient has a problem which needs sorting out. It may be grief, which requires giving the patient an ear to listen rather than a mouthful of instruments. Grief can be due to any loss, from the smashed up car, to the death of a loved one.

Grief is the pain of loss and we should be very concerned to understand how it relates to dentistry. Patients grieve over the loss of a tooth, over the loss of a smile, over the loss of comfort and confidence, over the loss of the ability to eat. Since any loss, however small, causes grief, however mild, we should (if we are responsible for it) help that patient over the experience, firstly by preparing them lovingly in advance, and secondly by helping them after the loss to come through to the end of the grief, which is acceptance and peace. The stages people go through (although not necessarily in this order) are as follows: numbness of mind, almost detachment, appearing to be completely unconcerned — this is usually the immediate reaction; refusal to believe it has happened; self criticism and blame (if only I hadn't done something the loss wouldn't have occurred); bargaining — (dear God, if you will just let me have it — him back, I will ...); questioning — why me? and finally, (but not always), anger. This is the one we dentists should be most aware of, as it can impinge directly on us. People get angry because they have suffered the loss and want to take it out on the dentist, or even very occasionally, the profession. Loren Pilling tells the story of a woman who actually made a hobby of going round dentists with a bag full of unsatisfactory dentures. She flattered the new dentist — surely he could succeed where others failed. Then she could revenge her loss of teeth by knocking the dentist down again. Eventually, she was suing six dentists at the same time. Love helps here, because one's concern will prompt a really thorough evaluation of the patient before doing anything, and seeing all those previous dentures in a bag must suggest that a number of colleagues have tried to help her in the past. She may need psychiatry rather than dentistry!

And as far as our other patients are concerned their visit is a time to try and understand the element of grief involved in what we are doing to them and to minimise its effect. Love demands no less.

Love also demands that we try and pick up depression at the earliest possible opportunity. We see patients regularly. Maybe we are the only medical advisers who do have access to patients on such a regular basis over a life time. We can see that something is different with patients since their last check-up. With depression the real key is loss of interest; it is the real sign that the patient is depressed and we can do something about it, by talking to, or rather listening to the patient, and by contacting the relatives. Again, it may be right to suggest that a good psychiatrist might help.

Love is even more all-embracing than this. It demands that we go out and spread it around the world. The 'actualised' person, the achiever, will want to become involved in giving in many ways: give to the local community by being active in community affairs; join your church council or synagogue; join in your local party politics; help on local health bodies or school boards; help in dentistry by spreading knowledge and love; share your good things with the world. Your efforts will be repaid a hundred fold as people around you love you and each other more, and as more of your schemes, projects and ideas grow and bear fruit. And bear fruit they will, because love is active, not passive. Love achieves; love builds up; love brings peace and prosperity to all; love is everything that is worthwhile in the traditions of the great nations of the west. With love, all things bloom and become fruitful; without love, all is desolation, and hatred and destruction.

Always remember the sentiment expressed by the holy man from the desert, Carlo Caretto. 'When I cease to love I make myself unhappy. When I resent someone I know no peace. I eat my own heart out through sleepless nights which torment me and sap my energy'. I'm sure we have all had the experience of stopping loving someone and making ourselves miserable through our own resentment. Surely life is too short to fall into this trap.

Whether we like it or not, we are made for love. Love is the aim of our lives and the reason for our existence. It is the only thing capable of really satisfying me, and is the one thing which it is impossible to overdo.

7

Worship

In Britain, and to a large extent in Western Europe, worship is a discarded word. People affect to think it is not necessary any more and even to despise it. Why then is it so important? Why was it so important to Aristotle, and why has it been so important to countless generations over more than six thousand years of history? Why is worship so important to primitive tribes who have had no contact with the outside world for centuries? Why does the idea of worship persist in spite of powerful historical movements like the French Revolution, and in spite of strenuous efforts by socialist governments to stamp it out?

There are various matters related to these questions, but before considering them it is important to realise that it is not the purpose of this treatise to promote any sect or any type of religion. It is not necessary to have a religious affiliation to be philosophical and to try to understand and fulfil one's self. Having said that, it is also important to realise that religion has been the repository of philosophy for thousands of years, and that many of the best philosophical ideas will be found in religion. Since man does not seem to have changed much over the millennia, many of these ideas will still be relevant today, and may hopefully be discussed in a detached and unprejudiced way. Having grown to maturity in the western world, many of the ideas we come across in our society will be based in the Judaeo-Christian tradition.

Why Worship is Important

Let us discuss the point under separate headings. Firstly — everyone has a god — what or who is yours? Secondly, ones stance in relation to the universe in which we live. Thirdly, the powerful inbuilt desire to be part of eternity. Fourthly, the non-spiritual aspects of religion.

What or who is your god? We all have one, and yours is the idea or object which is the summit of your hopes and aspirations, your main inspiration and motive in life. For some people it is money; they have what St. Paul described as that love of money which makes a man an idolator. You all know someone like this, who is prepared to sacrifice himself (or herself) and his or her family at the altar of the god; keeping family in penury, and abusing staff with slave labour in order to please their god by amassing more wealth. The temptation is always there to cheat on business deals and to suppress weaker individuals for a little extra money. In dentistry it can result in resentment towards staff if they ask for decent wages, failure to spend enough money to keep up to date with knowledge and equipment, and worst of all, a temptation to try and get away with shoddy work, cutting corners in order to earn a little more for a smaller outlay. This last is a very real temptation with insurance schemes where the remuneration is on a piece-work basis by a fixed scale of fees. The more time and trouble taken by the dentist, the smaller the reward. In private contract dentistry the temptation is to overcharge the patients, or to try and sell unnecessary work. Remember the true philosophy, a fair fee is that which will enable the dentist to do his best work and which the patient will recognise as reasonable. This last will lead to an atmosphere of love, and in the end the dentist will do better than if he cheats. The god of money is a false god, and its worship leads to lack of self esteem, and bitterness with one's family, staff, and patients.

Then there is the god of self importance. Some people will do anything to curry favour with their fellow beings. Their pride is so great that flattery is welcome, however insincere. They end up paying dearly for this, since people know that a particular person can easily be used by manipulating his god. A few flattering words and the person is buying drinks and dinners. Then he may be led into putting up money for doubtful deals in exchange for doubtful promises of 'status' appointments. Again, these people tend to undermine their own happiness because they see their families as a responsibility which detracts from their own personal advancement, so they skimp on time and money spent on the family in order to spend more time and money currying the favour of unimportant strangers. This sort of person spends more time at the golf club bar, buying drinks in exchange for flattery than he does building up the real source of happiness in the home. Such friends as he finds at the bar are fair weather friends who melt away when times are hard and he no longer has the price of a few drinks to buy their flattery. How sharp their tongues can be then and what a harsh crash to earth awaits him. The social climber who has slipped is indeed a pathetic figure.

Other people have gods of materialism — possessions. It can be anything from a stamp collection to a country estate. I once knew a chap who skimped on the house-keeping and kept the family on the breadline just in order to save up and buy an expensive car. He made it in the end and I hope it brought him the pleasure he imagined it would. Since it was some years ago, the car is probably a rust heap now. I wonder just how he is making out with his wife and children? Did they forgive him? Has he made it up to them? Or are his children teenage strangers and his wife distant and estranged?

Is this the same fate that awaits the dentist who makes dentistry his god? Oh yes — we all know them, the workaholics who neglect everything else so that they can think dentistry all the time. What a good thing it is to strive for excellence, but how foolish to make it into a god.

Then think of hedonism. People make the good time, *la dolce vita*, their god. Fast women or gigolos, fast cars or jewelery, gambling and drinking, frequently combined with a desire to impress with all the latest fashions. Everything is dissipated in one endless round of merriment until all the substance of life is gone. And as one becomes accustomed to the thrill, then the thrill becomes cheap and ordinary, and one has to chase after more and more bizarre diversions! People end up in some very kinky and sordid backwaters. And what happens to their self esteem? Do you think they can really be happy when in their hearts they despise themselves? Lack of self esteem is one of the greatest causes of mental disease. What a false god that brings people to such depths of degradation.

So have a good look at yourself. What is your god (or gods — because it is possible to try to serve more than one)? In the end, surely you will want to serve the God of love, truth, justice and honour. As Abraham Maslow says, a desire for these things is an inbuilt part of our human state. In the hierarchy of needs, one starts with basic needs like air, water, food, warmth and shelter. When these needs have been satisfied, man reaches out for a whole hierarchy of spiritual desires such as love, belongingness and self esteem. When these needs have been satisfied, one looks for truth, goodness, beauty, justice, order, etc. These things are necessary in life for fulfilment. They are a part of our nature which has to be satisfied. It is no coincidence that these are also the aims of most of the religions of the world. And ultimately, it is only the realisation of these things which can bring peace and self actualisation to the spirit, which can bring individuals to healthy, happy and more effective lives. Conversely, frustration of these needs causes development of psycho-pathological symptoms.

The writer of the book of Ecclesiastes said it all three thousand years ago — all is vanity. He freely confessed he had tried every kind of god — from money and possessions to sexual delight and self aggrandisement. But he never really found peace until he found how he fitted into the great big wonderful world of creation. It is up to you to find out how you fit in too, and to come to terms with your place in the universe and your life and death if you would be happy. It does not matter whether you find help through one of the established sects, or if you do it privately. Ultimately, it is a personal thing for everyone because we are all unique. There has never been anyone exactly like you, and there never will be. As St. Thomas More said, 'no man can get to heaven on anyone else's back'. You have to do it for yourself in your own unique way. You may be a humanist, an agnostic, a Catholic, a Jew, a Buddhist or a Moslem. Of course, being part of an established sect helps because you will meet like-minded people who are all pulling in the same direction. Thus you help to strengthen each others resolve and deepen each others understanding. The problem of being a 'loner' is that the going gets very tough when the temptations to weakness are strong. And we have seen that self discipline is an extremely important thing. It is easy to modify one's ideal to accommodate a temptation if there is no sheet anchor to hold on to. But if you have the self discipline to do it, then good luck to you. To know where you are in this great big wonderful world and to come to terms with your relation to life and death, that is the important thing.

Worship in Society

But what about worship in relation to the society in which we live? Society has its gods, too. They are the summation of what the majority of people think, combined with the strength of will of those individuals in pursuing their own god. It is like a crowd in a swimming pool. If one section combines together to splash others and they do it with all their strength, they will be able to command the most comfortable part of the pool, the shallow end. The others will be pushed into the deep end. Then the weaker members in the deep end will change sides and go with the ones in the shallow end for the sake of an easy time. If the people in the deep end do not splash back with all their vigour then they will be pushed into a more untenable position where their feet cannot touch the bottom and they will either drown or have to leave the pool, or only stay with greatest difficulty. If only they had made a greater effort earlier on they need not have been pushed out. It is the same in society. In any social group, large or small, all that is necessary for evil to triumph is for good people to do nothing. The same applies to nations, and even to the world.

If the majority of people have hedonism for their god, they will be so busy chasing the good time that they will not notice people with evil gods working to dominate society. And in chasing the god of pleasure at all costs, they will have thrown away the real good things, such as justice, honour, truth and virtue. This is how societies come to be dominated by false gods. International socialism is a case in point.

Socialism is atheistic. Marx begins his book *Das Kapital* with the famous words 'There is no God. Therefore there is no after life. Religion is the opiate of the people'. This immediately sets the Socialistic state apart as something different from most of the states of the western world, which have been based on a Christian ideal. The Western tradition has been that first comes the God of truth, justice, virtue, honour and the ten commandments. Since this is so, these ideals permeate our society and we expect to be treated with justice, and in an honourable way. Next in the hierarchy comes man, unique and individualistic, with freedom of the will. This gives everyone dignity and a place in society. Thirdly comes the state, which is a collection of individuals and families gathered together for their mutual benefit. Thus the state is the servant of the individual and freedom of the citizen is preserved.

Compare this with the socialist system. International socialism is the Socialists' God, and comes first in their hierarchy. Secondly comes the socialist state which is subservient to the international socialist ideal. Lastly comes the individual citizen who is subservient to the state and 'the party'. Once you have understood this, then the difference between their society and ours is easy to comprehend. Because International Socialism is God then what is good for it is paramount; and since the god of justice and truth has been toppled over, then there is no need to act in accordance with these virtues. Indeed Marx and Engels have made it quite clear that the good socialist must not only be prepared to crawl on his belly in the dust if needs be, but must also be ready to cheat, lie, steal or kill in the cause of international socialism. Socialism is a jealous god, and brooks no opposition. There is no justice as we know it in their courts of law, and terrible imprisonments, torturings and executions are administered in the name of their brand of 'justice'. And one has to be extremely careful in any dealing with them as they cannot be relied on to tell the truth. They will always say or do that which seems at the moment to offer the best advantage to their God, international socialism. This indeed *is* their morality, the pursuit of international socialism without any pretence to truth or virtue as we know it. Why? Because they worship a false god.

If you wish to live in a society which will respect individual rights and the rights of the family, then you must make things like justice and truth your god, and you must be prepared to go out and work for them in your community. Work for them in your club, on your child's school parent/teacher association, on your local political committees, in your profession, in your family and above all in yourself. Do not be put off by the thought that one person cannot achieve very much. It is better to light *one* candle than to curse the darkness. A certain philosopher used to illustrate this point by having all the lights put out in the hall in which he was speaking. Then he would strike a match on stage. The effect of one match was quite amazing. Then he asked people in this audience to light their cigarette lighters. The result was a blaze of light throughout the whole auditorium. All the good and bad things in this world have been started by just one person, and sustained by others following on. So if you want personal peace, you must choose the right gods for yourself and if you want a decent society then you should pursue this with great energy. Let your little light shine. Be a doer, not just a hearer.

But is that enough? We have seen that in order to be happy we have to come to terms with death; death of our loved ones, and death for ourselves. This is not a sordid subject to be swept under the carpet. It is a fact of life. The one thing we all know is that we are going to die. We have to make our peace with this knowledge one way or another. Many people can live quite comfortably with the idea that death is the end of all things. Others find this more difficult. They see the great universe and feel that being part of this must include more than our life span on earth. Indeed an appreciation of some idea of eternity seems to be part of the makeup of man, since it continually appears in all sorts of societies around the world, from sophisticated societies to primitive isolated groups. In the twelfth century, St. Thomas Aquinas defined eternity as a never ending present. Now, thanks to Einstein's theory of relativity every schoolboy knows that a spaceman who was accelerated to the speed of light would exist in a never ending present, because time would stand still for him. As the French say, '*Toujours les mêmes choses*'!! So it is possible to get outside time. And since the 'Big Bang' and the 'Steady State' theories of the origin of the universe both rely on creation, then it is possible to envisage a creator who exists outside of our time span, some being who possesses existence as of a right and can bestow it on our universe. Is it a coincidence that the word Jehova means 'I am who am'? And what is our universe anyway? When physicists examine the smallest elements they find no substance, only energy. St. Thomas Aquinas said that God maintains creation in existence from moment to moment, and that if he did not, it would revert back to nothing. If the energy of the universe was suddenly withdrawn, then

St. Thomas could well be right. If the energy of the universe is like light, then truly the creator would be the God of Light and away from him all would be darkness. But more important, if the creator is the God of Love, then all around him will be love. Away from him there would be no love. Surely this would be hell! Hell on earth is surely to live in a loveless condition of our own making. As the Bhudda said, we certainly make our own heaven or hell on this earth, according to the gods we choose. Even in the adversity of the concentration camps there were people who carried heaven in their hearts, and they were not afraid of death. Somehow we have to emulate them, to love; and to work even under the most horrific conditions to promote love in the world. This is surely the point about worship, to love, and to attain union with creation, to make a heaven on earth through working for justice and truth and virtue, and to prepare ourselves for death in the knowledge that we have fulfilled ourselves through the realisation of everything that is best in our own unique nature. Then according to the Bhudda we will be absorbed into Nirvanah, into creation itself — peace and love. According to Judaeo-Christianity, we can expect to be taken up into heaven to the ultimate fulfilment of seeing and knowing the creator in all his wonder and glory, for all eternity. For Moslems, the goal is similar, attainment of paradise with Allah.

So there we have it. Worship is important. And if we would be happy and fulfilled then we should sort out which gods we serve, and which gods we want to serve. A simple question of sorting out our priorities and making a plan. Know where you are in the great big wonderful world. Without coming to terms with these things you will not find inner *peace or fulfilment* in this life, never mind the next!

Worship in the Practice

Most of us will not be content to just think about worship. We will want to actually do something to fulfil this need in our nature in a charitable way. Charity is a word meaning love in its highest sense, but the word has become debased into meaning just doing charitable works. The important thing is to realise that good deeds are really only the physical expression of the love and awareness of one's involvement with others on this earth. For dentists this aspect all fits into the worship arm of the cross of life (See chapter I). It fulfils the need to give something back for all the gifts we have been given. For some people it will be treating certain patients in a charitable way. Some dentists treat orphans, or the old and handicapped for minimal fees or even for free. Others write articles or books for no reward, or donate the royalties to charity. Other people work outside the profession, helping on the board of a local charity, or even just collecting clothes or money, or organising fund-raising events. There are so many practical outlets of this kind and opportunities abound! They do not have to be sought, they are self evident. Whatever it is, if you feel you want to become involved, then don't hesitate, do it.

❦8❦

Work

Work should be one of the most satisfying things in this life. In dentistry we are lucky, because we work in a profession which offers limitless opportunities to fill a lifetime with interest, and wonder, and pleasure of achievement.

But work is not only a pleasure, it is a necessity for physical and mental health. We all need to feel we are useful in this world. Dislike for oneself and recognition that one's life is being wasted are two of the failings of humanity according to Abraham Maslow. And if maturity is being fully human, and mental illness a falling away from fullness of humanity, then lack of self respect and meaningfulness in life are two of the great factors which undermine mental health. We all need to think that we are worthwhile, and are making a valuable contribution in the world. A well loved member of my family retired from a lifetime's work in a large business organisation. Immediately he became most unhappy and he even diagnosed the cause of his unhappiness very accurately. He said he felt suddenly worthless and unnecessary because he wasn't doing a meaningful job and making his usual valuable contribution. No one came up to him any more to ask how to do things, or where the details for certain processes could be obtained. His general health went rapidly downhill and in six months he was dead! It was said at the time that he died of boredom, but in fact he died because he had been deprived of meaningful work and had been unable to nourish his real, deep psychological need with hobbies such as gardening, charitable works or some other worthwhile occupation. He disliked himself because he felt that from now on he would be a worthless member of society, and that any skills and knowledge he had built up would henceforth be wasted! This is one of the great problems with retirement, and explains why so many people, particularly those with few hobbies, do not live long when they retire.

So work is necessary for all of us. But it has to be meaningful work. People working at boring repetitive jobs tend to develop neuroses because their work lacks meaning and they think their lives are being wasted. One extremely helpful approach was discovered by Elton Mayo from the Harvard Graduate School of Business Administration. He found that by involving the workers in simple decisions such as the optimum level of lighting, or optimum length of rest periods, they found importance, meaning and status, and their work and productivity improved. They became worthwhile in their own eyes and so they wanted to give the best account of themselves. And they felt happier and more fulfilled when they went home at night.

Dentists as Workers

Dentists are human just like any other workers. And most of them have an additional advantage; they are their own boss. Alas! Too many do not take advantage of this, but allow themselves to work in depressing surroundings and in a style and manner which encourages boring repetitiveness. So many dentists are unhappy and unfulfilled because they are not prepared to escape from the trap of doing nothing but boring, simple repetitive repair work and destructive 'blood and acrylic' style dentistry which destroys their sense of self worth. They have given themselves a psychosis by being their own bad and inconsiderate employer. And to cap it all they blame dentistry for their unhappy state. One dentist told me that dentistry was not comprehensive enough to fulfil him, and that he felt he should have been a brain surgeon. I thought to myself he would have made just as lousy a brain surgeon as he did a dentist because his whole attitude of mind was wrong and that was the root of the problem. With his mental attitude he would have had great difficulty turning the presidency of the U.S.A. into a meaningful job of work! Dentistry is *so* worthwhile if we will only open our minds to the possibilities!

Think for a moment about the variety of satisfaction to be obtained from dentistry. First and most important is the choice of employment. Dentists can choose to work for an institution such as a hospital, or the armed forces, or to be employed by a large firm. And these institutions and firms can offer great opportunities to travel and see the world, even to work in a foreign country for long periods of time. But most important of all is the opportunity to be one's own employer.

The opportunity to be self employed is good because it offers such scope for fulfilment. One can choose how and where to practice and with whom. And how many people have the chance to choose exactly who they will work with? The self employed dentist can even choose his patients, because he has the power to refuse any patient if he wishes to do so. He can even decide which aspects of dentistry he will undertake and which he will refer to other practitioners. And by 'he' I mean 'you', the dentist reading this page! You can work in the climate of your choice, in the neighbourhood or the town of your choice,

with the staff of your choice, and on the patients that you
choose, doing the kind of work that you like. You can work
what hours you want to, and take holidays and time off just
when you decide. And you can work in surroundings that
you find attractive and in an interior decor that appeals to
you. And most important of all you can change these
things as you wish. It is not necessary to continue to work
as you have been doing if your family circumstances or
objectives change, or if you fancy something different. You
can change it; yes, YOU! You can rebuild the inside of
your practice, or even move to another address, maybe in
another town or even another state. I know of one dentist
in Britain who completely transformed his practice from
an all National Health basic 'filling station' type of
practice into an exclusive all private contract practice by
simply moving into another house not 200 yards away
from his former abode. That move was his act of
commitment. This is very important, to do something as a
definite gesture to mark the turning point. With Dr.
Pankey it was his commitment never to extract another
tooth. But for you it could be anything from buying a new
carpet to symbolically burning your insurance contract!
Satisfying and meaningful work is necessary for the soul,
and such a big part of mental health that it is important to
get it right. Don't just sit and grumble, do something.
Remember you are free; you are unique; you are the
master of your fate and the captain of your soul, so go out
and realise your own uniqueness. Be self actualising, make
yourself into an actuality, a reality, instead of just a
shadow of what you might have been.

Improving the image of one's practice is the gateway to
so much more fulfilment. Immediately the possibility of
more interesting and fulfilling work opens up. And don't
just think of the technical side of dentistry, think of the

artistic opportunities that present themselves. Even a simple amalgam filling can be a thing of beauty, and just to run a mirror round a really clean and healthy mouth is a joyous and most aesthetically pleasing thing. And with super crowns and bridges, it is not just the technical beauty, or the aesthetic qualities of the porcelain, but the beauty of the super pink gum sitting all happy and healthy around the tooth which satisfies. Surely it is true that the beauty of the soft tissues reflects the excellence of dentistry. And above all the minutae of beauty, is the satisfaction of helping to create an attractive smile, and to contribute to the building up of a beautiful and confident personality in your patient.

Artistic fulfilment does not stop with aesthetics. As a dentist, one can fulfil oneself in so many other ways. Every job is done before a small audience, the patient and the nurse, and so becomes a performance as on a stage. Then there is the impact of the work on relatives and friends. The mouths of our patients should be like mobile art galleries carrying our beautiful sculptures to a wider audience. What pleasure, what satisfaction, what fulfilment, to complete worthwhile dentistry and know how many people in the world will benefit from the beauty, and confident smiles they see! And this is only part of the opportunity for artistic expression which the profession offers. One can work on a wider stage by showing one's work at study groups and on table clinics. And one can go even further to an audience: actually giving a performance on a stage! How many times have you regretted that a dental lecturer did not realise that he needed at least some knowledge of theatre to project his lecture in a meaningful and interesting way? Making crowns and dentures may be just a three-dimensional sculptural exercise — but the preparation of slides to illustrate it is an aesthetic exercise in two-dimensional artistry. And if your need of artistic expression extends to writing, why then the opportunities are endless. You can write articles for the dental press, and even for the local press. The articles can be technical, humorous, or of general interest (travel, holidays, etc.). A friend of mine even manages to write articles on cars for a dental publication, and has created for himself the opportunity of driving all the latest models. He conceived, he believed and he achieved! And they call this work! To most people the opportunity to achieve all this artistic expression is heaven, and for most of them just about as far away. Dentists have a pearl of great price in their hand, an object for which many people would sell all their other possessions. Many dentists however might as well throw it away with the garbage. They do not seem to realise its existence, much less its worth.

There is another immensely enjoyable factor in dentistry and that is the creativity of working to the highest standards, and of rebuilding people's mouths into a health promoting state. The engineering skills required are vaired, demanding and extremely satisfying when put to good use. It is a world of its own, and yet a microcosm of all major engineering work, with decisions as to how and where to absorb stresses and strains, and to create a beautiful and functional end product. And above our engineering skills we have extra challenges to overcome, because we are not just dealing with mechanics as most engineers are, but with bio-mechanics; and this adds an extra fascination and a new dimension.

The Rewards

I have not even touched on the other exciting aspects of dentistry, the healing of disease, the removal of pain, the surgical skills, the joy of actually working with one's hands and brain and having an end product. Really there is so much joy and satisfaction I feel we should paraphrase Robert Louis Stevenson and say that 'Dentistry is so full of such wonderful things I think we should all be as happy as kings!' And just think, it goes on for a whole lifetime too!! There is always something new to learn, and new standards of excellence to aspire to. Dentistry is a fascinating job which can be done even in old age, and in which the interest need never flag. No wonder some dentists find it difficult to keep in balance. And yet this must be done. All work and no play makes Jack a dull boy. It is pointless to work all day and neglect other aspects of life. Time must be found for love, and for one's family. One's family is paramount and in the end work exists as a means of supporting it. Do not fall into the trap of working so hard that you give your family all the material things but never have time to be with them or to show them your love. If material things are all that you give them you cannot expect love in return. Remember love begets love. And you cannot bring love into your practice and your work and ignore it in your family, the very heart of your life. Give some thought to worship, to your fellow beings and to where you are in relation to the rest of creation. Balance is so important.

Of course, life can be (perhaps has to be) out of balance for a short period. It is most often in the early days of business that one may have to spend extra time at work in order to build up and establish oneself, but this must be recognised and one's plan should envisage an end to the period of imbalance; which should be as short as possible.

9

Play

A great many dentists seem to have a puritanical ethic. As a profession we seem to think that it is almost sinful to enjoy ourselves, and the feeling persists that if we are not working, we can't be up to much good! As a result, our lives get out of balance. We never really fulfil ourselves because we do not give enough time to developing those aspects of play — travel, art, music, sport or even quiet contemplative relaxation — which are so important. As Abraham Maslow points out, playfulness is one of the attributes of the 'self-actualised' man. And since a proper appreciation of play in life is a characteristic of all the most mentally healthy, most successful and fulfilled people in the world, then surely it is something which we should all acquire. Just as we have to find time for work, for fostering love in our families, and for worship, so we have to find time for recreation.

Fortunately, we are all different, and all of us are uniquely qualified to find the type and style of play which fits in with our own character and needs. Some people are participators and others are spectators. Most of us are a mixture of both. Many people who would rather play in a game than watch it would also be much happier in an audience at the theatre than acting on the stage. And the reverse is equally true. Some people enjoy contact sport, others cannot bear it. Some like to be part of a team, others to do their own thing. Many like to be part of a crowd, others like solitude. One woman I know who enjoyed holidays in crowded resorts could not understand her daughter who chose to go somewhere quiet for the vacation. So it is up to each one of us to decide what we would like to do in our own way and make provision to bring this into the balance of our lives. It is no sin to be happy. It is no sin to enjoy oneself. There is nothing wrong in enjoying the fruits of one's labours, and providing one's family with the good things of life. Indeed, these things are to be encouraged since it is the promise of reward which sweetens labour. If one is prosperous as a result of hard work and early sacrifice, one has earned the rewards. There should be no conscientious scruples about this.

Play has two aspects: those which are connected with the home, and those which are outside the home circle. And under both these headings are two subdivisions, those which we do with the family and those which are done alone.

Play and the Family

We have already discussed the importance of the home and the family. There is nothing which gives more lasting joy and pleasure and true happiness than a good family life. Forget the 'knockers' and the 'libertarians' and do not be put off by cruel jibes about being staid or cabbage-like. Make your home and marriage the centre of your life. And sexual satisfaction is all part of a good marriage. True sexual maturity is in finding lasting and continuing happiness through a lifetime with the same marriage partner. People who have a series of extra-marital affairs, 'one night stands', or 'quickie' sexual encounters are really advertising their own sexual immaturity to the world. They are not mature enough to make a lasting relationship. They are also advertising their immaturity in their unfaithfulness, deceit, selfishness and irresponsibility. The sort of play which encourages immorality is destructive of self, of home and of family and should be avoided. Mature married couples have a much more rewarding sex life because they can explore each other's personality and physique to the full, and in their depth of knowledge of themselves and their marriage partner they can find heights of fulfilment far beyond the understanding of a casual encounter. It is very pertinent that Abraham Maslow found successful and lasting marriage to be one of the characteristics of self-actualised people. A good marriage is not only satisfying and fulfilling, but it builds up positive self respect and provides that stability and security which is necessary for one's own growth towards maturity. It also forms the foundation for healthy growth and development of one's children's personalities. Good family life also provides the basis for a happy and rewarding experience in later life, when one can watch one's children applying the philosophy they have been taught, and bringing their children to their grandparents, for the pleasure of all.

Within the family there are endless opportunities for play, both as a family unit and also as pairs of individuals. It is important to try to understand one's children, since more heartbreak has been caused because parents did not realise that their children did not automatically enjoy the same sort of recreation as themselves than for any other reason. It is natural for parents who were good at ball games to hope their children will be so as well, but it does not necessarily follow, and be to be forced into an activity which one detests is purgatory for a child. What a terrible conflict between their loyalty to their parents and their abhorrence of the particular pastime which the parents hold dear! You must seek to 'know your children' just as you 'know yourself' and 'know your patient'. Then it is possible to find some form of recreation which is acceptable to both parent and child. There is such a wide range of activities from music, singing, dancing and painting, to active sports, both solo games and team games. Respect the child's nature and character and show parental maturity by seeking out the areas of play you will both appreciate. Look also for things which can be enjoyed as a family unit, always trying to find time for the family to do things together. And use your earnings to provide pleasant surroundings and an opportunity for play at home. Get that swimming pool, or tennis court; buy that boat, or paddock for the horse; build that music room, if that is what the family want, and then enjoy it together.

But do not forget that everyone also needs those periods of quiet. We all require some time for solitude, and this should be available to us in the home; other people's solitude should be respected. It is also possible to go out alone either for some activity like a quiet walk through the countryside, or just climbing up into a tree for a little quiet reflection and contemplation. Many adults find this through activities such as fishing or even just walking up to the top of a hill and enjoying the view. Find time for this aspect of play.

Other Aspects of Play

Reading is another aspect of play. It can be very educational and one can choose reading matter in a positive way, to encourage one's mind to grow in a beneficial direction. Remember, we do not have to let other people influence us in ways we do not want. (Don't let them write on *your* sheet of paper!) So be choosy. And do not simply read to educate the mind; spend a little time reading entertaining trivia. If you like cowboy novels, then read them. This is better than sitting mindlessly in front of the television. TV is not necessarily bad; but be selective.

Travel is also an important aspect of play. Seeing the way other nations live, and how other cultures cope with the problems of life broadens the mind and helps to create deeper understanding. It also offers opportunities to spend some time in different climates and geographical surroundings and to enjoy sports which would not be possible in one's home country. There is also the opportunity to see different styles of architecture, to hear music and see paintings and sculptures which are quite different from those at home. All these things are rewarding and enriching. And the interesting thing is how happy people are to come back to their homes. A spell in a different country certainly makes one appreciate one's own environment and one's own home.

Finally, do not forget the principle of balance. Our 'cross' can be out of balance through concentration on 'play' just as much as over-concentration on the other basic needs. I know one chap who is mad on golf. I'm sure his golf swing is his god. He spends so much time on the golf course his family hardly know him, and he is now taking extra time off from business to play golf. He wonders why he is unhappy! But a few extra hours on the golf course are unlikely to put things right. His neglect of the other parts of life has made him so unhappy that it seems that he is only happy with a golf club in his hand. But the true answer would be for him to spend more time on the other aspects of life. If he devoted as much time to love, work and worship as he does to his golf, he would not only resolve his problems, but would create positive happiness for himself and those close to him. Happiness is not all just luck. It is something which can be positively worked for. And when it comes, it should be recognised. One of the most difficult things in life is to be able to say 'Now I am happy!' Play your cards right and you will be.

10

Health

In my youth, the ideal was to have a healthy mind in a healthy body. It was a fine ideal then and is a fine ideal now. Baden Powell based his philosophy of scouting on the idea. A healthy mind is a happy mind and the object of this book has been to follow the mental approach to happiness in dentistry. But there are other aspects of life which press severely upon dentists and which will cause great unhappiness if they are not recognised and tackled early on. In order to be happy we should consider various aspects of health, eg., our general health, our own dental health, the health of our practice, and our financial health. If we can build into our lives an understanding of the importance of these things then we will end up achieving health and wealth as well as happiness.

To begin with, let us look at our own health. It is obviously necessary to be healthy. We all want to avoid illness. But is this negative approach enough? The answer must be a firm NO. Our minds and bodies are like any other machine, they run better when they are well looked after and properly maintained. Dentistry is a very demanding profession and it is necessary to be in good physical shape if we are to cope with the stresses and strains to which we are subjected. There is an old adage about physical prowess — use it or lose it! It is very true. We need to exercise and keep fit in order that our bones and muscles will be able to cope with the stress of bending over all day and spending long periods of time in a tiring position. Many dentists end up with back troubles through neglecting to keep their backs supple and strong through adequate exercise, and through failing to understand the importance of exercise movements during the working day. This neglect can lead to severe problems which may well involve several weeks away from work whilst they are resolved, with consequent stress and worry associated with the loss of income. All this can be avoided with proper exercise which can, and should, be an enjoyable and relaxing pastime. Exercise can be partaken in solitude or in company, and the company can be either family or friends. When we share the enjoyment of exercise we not only build up our own health, but we build up relationships, and deepen friendships and family ties.

It is important to realise that physical health affects mental performance. Which of us has not had the experience of being physically 'out of sorts' and finding that it was difficult to concentrate the mind on the job in hand or to make decisions. This is true in the dental surgery, and when we are 'one degree under' the alternative means of treating the same problem do not spring so readily to mind. In addition, our general life and demeanour are depressed by poor physical health; we become more irritable and more inclined to look on the gloomy side of things. Conversely, physical fitness leads to a healthy, more relaxed mind, which works efficiently and is happy. Small irritations are easily overcome with a smile instead of a scowl, and it is great to feel on top of things both at home and at work. So physical fitness is very important to us and we should set about achieving it in a safe and enjoyable way.

We should take account of both enjoyment and the safety. We are all unique and for that reason we all enjoy different things. Therefore we have to search for some sort of physical sport or exercise which appeals to us. We need not overdo it, and reasonable fitness can be obtained with minimal effort. We are not all training to represent our country at sport, and there is no need to go about our exercise programme as if we were. So choose a simple and attractive form of exercise suited to your particular desires, age group, physical ability etc., and go about it sensibly.

True Fitness

The best athletes and most knowledgeable physical fitness instructors will not attempt to participate in an un-accustomed sport unless they have done a few relevant exercises. One friend of mine, for example, refused to play a friendly game of tennis at a country house weekend, because he understood the risks of strained and pulled muscles, which can happen when they are suddenly called upon to function at much higher stress levels than they are accustomed to. This was in spite of the fact that he was very fit, and an excellent performer at his own sport. We should all learn a lesson from him and start any new exercise programme gradually, with an eye to our age and general physical condition. Start with the simplest of exercises and gradually build up stamina over a long period. There is no hurry, and it is better to be a bit overcautious than to rush into something and later regret it. It is also good to have a thorough physical check up with one's doctor before embarking on a course of exercise. Better safe than sorry. And follow a programme by someone who really knows what he is talking about. For example, Dr Cooper wrote a book on Aerobics, and Lawrence Moorehouse and Leonard Gross have written 'Total fitness in 30 minutes a week'.

But fitness is more than exercise. Physically we are the product of the food we eat. If we supply our bodies with a good and sufficient diet we can expect to promote fitness. If we abuse ourselves by over-eating, or eating the wrong foods, we are poisoning ourselves and predisposing ourselves to disease. Our attitude toward our bodies should be similar to our objective for our patients; to encourage health. The body needs to be healthy; that is its object in life. If we encourage it to be healthy it will respond. A good diet is therefore desirable.

All diets should be regarded as guidelines, not lists of unbreakable commandments. Occasionally it is good to have a party and enjoy rich food and wine, but for most of the time it is good to train our palates and our stomachs to enjoy a sufficiency of wholesome health giving fare.

Fitness is not just a product of exercise and diet. It is also concerned with stress levels and environment. There is mounting evidence that stress promotes disease. The more stress that one has to undergo the more one's physical health deteriorates; and if people are subjected to stress over a certain level, then one can almost predict that severe physical disease will follow. This stress may be something outside of our control, such as the death of a loved one, but stress can also be self-inflicted; and the whole point of this philosophy is to try and live one's life in a way which will promote happiness and health by diminishing unnecessary stress. It is important to remember that stress feeds upon itself. If we are in a stressful situation our health and physical performance deteriorates and we are more inclined to make mistakes, which cause more stress. Then one accident tends to follow another. It is not a coincidence. The later accidents are the result of diminished ability and performance levels caused by the previous accident. There are two possible solutions; firstly to live as much as possible in a way which can cope with the stresses of one's life style; secondly one should keep one's body in good physical shape, so that it is better able to resist the physical effect of stress.

Financial Health

Financial troubles are among the greatest stresses we may have to bear. If we cannot make ends meet we are in trouble. There are of course times when we all have to put ourselves in debt; financing our practice, and buying a house are the two most common. But many dentists are extremely imprudent and try to run before they can walk financially. They then find they have bought 'fun things' and 'status symbols' and burdened themselves with debts which they have difficulty in financing. They have not cut their coats according to the amount of cloth they have available, and as a result they are financially unhealthy. It is important to try and build up an understanding of the hierarchy of needs and demands on our financial resources. There are so many things we can live without for a time and if we use our common sense we will only be denying outselves these things for a short time.

Firstly, the greatest investment any dentist can make is in his knowledge of his work. Nothing will give a finer return on financial outlay than this. It begins at the dental school, but it should not stop just because we now have a few letters after our names. There are always new areas of knowledge to be explored, and dentists should continually strive to improve their knowledge and deepen their understanding by going on courses, joining study groups, attending conferences, and reading. The resultant keeping up with the best there is will be reflected in one's practice. One will attract the sort of patients who want the best treatment and are prepared to pay for it, and the financial return will far outstrip the original financial investment.

The next most important investment for any dentist is in the tools of his trade. This covers not only the instruments necessary to do the work but the premises and the way they are furnished and decorated. So make sure that you have good equipment and have back up facilities available in case anything goes wrong. In our practice, for example, we have a standby electricity generator and two air compressors. It may sound extravagant, but the price of an extra compressor is no more than the value of a couple of hours of lost turnover by the three dentists who work here; and think of the problem and embarrassment of cancellations and rescheduling of patients caused by a break down. In our practice the flick of a switch restores working ability in a moment. We also have an ample supply of spare handpieces, sterilisers and similar items. The most common 'economy' which is practised in a surprisingly large number of surgeries is the persistence in the use of carbide and diamond burs when they are well past their prime. It is no joy to the patient if a crown preparation takes twice as long because the diamonds are blunt, and the extra time also places an added stress on the dentist. Patients are not only aware of care taken and attention to detail but they are also well aware when things are moving smoothly and efficiently. And efficiency also extends to the ready availability of supplies. There should always be at least two spare packets of most things and there should be a reliable system of re-ordering. There is nothing more distressing than being half way through a proedure and then being unable to finish because some everyday item of supply is not in the stock cupboard. So do invest in good equipment and instruments and maintain them well, and institute a good inventory and reordering system.

Do not forget that the equipment also extends to the office, and that your staff will work better and more efficiently if they are well equipped and properly organised. This in turn will ensure that stress on the dentist is minimised. And staff extend to technical services. Your laboratory should be well equipped, and if you are obliged to use a commercial laboratory, make sure that you choose one that is well equipped, and pay enough for them to be able to give you back-up work of a standard that will complement what you are trying to do in the surgery. All these investments will help your practice to run smoothly and efficiently and to be more productive. In the long term they will amply repay their cost and the small effort necessary to organise them. Of course, you will not be able to buy all the most expensive equipment immediately, but it will come in time. At the beginning you must buy the most functional equipment your money will allow. But this does not mean that it should not look clean and artistic also. Remember the appearance of your practice is a reflection of yourself and if it looks a mess, then people are going to get an impression that to some extent they will be getting poor dentistry. Beauty and function usually go together. Make sure your practice reflects an image of the harmony between efficiency and aesthetics which you wish to achieve in people's mouths.

Having invested in one's knowledge, and in the 'tools of one's trade' it is then very important to protect that investment over the first crucial few years. The beginning of any business venture is always a critical time financially. Both capital investment and running costs must be considered. There will probably be rent to pay in advance not only for buildings, but for the other services like telephone etc. And then there will be staff wages to pay. For the first few months the work will very likely be scarce, and patients may well not want to pay until completion. This means that all the costs of running the business will have to be paid for about three months before money starts coming in. You will also want to eat during this period so a suitable arrangement must be made with the bank for adequate financial back up.

It is important to try and get into good habits in regard to 'cash flow' right from the beginning. This is the heart of good business management and it is vital to know just how one is faring in this respect. In our practice we have the precise financial position worked out at least twice a week, on Tuesday and Thursday. This is *not* based on the bank statement but on an accurate assessment of *ALL* the cheques which have either been signed or are awaiting signature. This way one does not come up with any nasty surprises. Large bills are all taken into account at the earliest possible moment, and money set aside for them. So do have a system which shows you exactly where you stand. You will also quickly realise the importance of getting the money in. Do not be sentimental about this; you are in business, you deserve to be paid for the service you give, and so you should be. Any delay means that, by financing the patient, you are losing the interest which would otherwise accrue and eventually being paid in money worth less than it was when you did the work, due to inflation. If inflation is running at 12% per annum this means that one month's delay is equivalent to a drop in value of 1%. If inflation is at 18% then this works out at $1\frac{1}{2}$% per month, or getting on for 5% when compounded over a three month period. And if interest rates are running at a similar level you could lose a similar amount through 'lost interest'. Can you really afford to be so generous to your patients as to lose around 9% of your fee because you were slack over sending accounts? It is important for patients to understand their financial responsibility right from the start. For simple treatment it is better that they pay by the visit *at the visit*. This saves them the problem of a big bill mounting up, and you have the money. For treatment spread over long periods of time terms of payment should be arranged BEFOREHAND so that the patient is aware that they will be required to pay instalments, and when the next instalments will fall due. It is helpful to write these figures down and have the patient initial them if in any doubt, or at least have your nurse initial the record card that these were the figures quoted. This precaution is usually unnecessary in a well run practice, since the patients will pay with gratitude; but there will always be an occasional case of misunderstanding or forgetfulness.

These arrangements will not necessarily apply to very rich class 1 patients who require special treatment, or to class 2 patients who need extensive work done. In the latter case it may be worthwhile to work out some means of paying the account by instalments, a sort of budget plan. The plan can be set up to fit in with the patient's needs, but I would like to see several payments made before work is commenced to build up a suitable capital sum, so that the arrangement can benefit both the dentist and the patient with regard to inflation and interest.

Financing capital expenses, and keeping an eye on cash flow will gradually reap its reward and the provident dentist who has lived simply and built up his business will begin to find that he has accumulated some capital. He can now begin to act like a successful man. The first investment he should make outside the business is in his own home.

This is most rewarding and the most necessary, because it encompasses the stability of the family and the extension of the love arm of Aristotle's Cross of Life. Not only will it promote family unity and stability but will also be a first class capital investment. As affluence increases, and the effects of knowing one's work and one's patients filter through, the house can be used as a stepping stone to more luxurious homes.

When the business and home are secure the next item for consideration will be one's children's future. It is good to make provision at the earliest time for the continuing education of one's family, not forgetting that they may want to go to university. Many insurance companies provide suitable policies. Find yourself a good insurance agent at an early date. (There will probably be one among your patients) and get good advice, on this and other things, such as family health provisions, business cover, personal and accident cover for self and spouse etc.

With continuing success one will find that there is more. money available. What should be done with this? Well, of course, there is always the love arm of Aristotle's cross, and some of this money should be used for charitable purposes. It is prudent, having done this, to use the surplus for a capital investment programme. Investments should help other people indirectly, and are therefore charitable acts. As long as you don't simply hoard money, whatever other use you put it to must benefit the community and other people. If you buy expensive toys like quality cars or boats then you are providing employment in those industries and in their distribution services. If you travel you are providing jobs in the travel industries. The same applies to any purchase, from hi-fi equipment and furniture to paintings or hand thrown pottery. Even expensive clothes have to be made and marketed and a large number of people rely on their sale for employment, right from the sheep shearer who produces expensive wool to the person who models the clothes. So any purchase helps many people in all sorts of ways. In addition, some of the tax paid on these items may go for social security payments to less fortunate members of society and to government sponsored overseas aid. The more tax you pay the higher your contribution. This is in addition to whatever charitable acts you may be carrying out on your own initiative.

Again, you can invest your money on the stock market. This is providing capital for business, and is also helping thousands of employees by providing jobs. In Britain one can invest in building societies which help other people to buy their own home, surely a worthy thing to do. Then there are insurances. Taking out insurance provides employment in the insurance industry, and also makes available funds for the insurance company to invest in other business ventures giving even more employment opportunities for working people. This argument could be extended indefinitely, but the fact is that it is very difficult to do something with money which does not help somebody else.

Management of money should involve some form of investment for the future. The love arm of Aristotle's cross demands that one provides not only for present needs of one's family but for the future as well. Most people should have a regular sum invested with the bank, or the building society or in some safe form of government stock. This is a good immediate reserve which is liquid enough to be easily available when required. In some countries like the U.S.A. this is a fantastically profitable investment if just left for the interest to accumulate at compound rates, and regular saving over the period of one's professional life would build up enough capital to be able to live on easily in one's retirement. In other countries like Britain tax is such that the benefit is much less apparent and it is advisable to think in terms of endowment insurance which has certain tax advantages, or pension policies. This latter should not be used with one's immediate reserves as the money can be frozen until the redeemable date, and may only be obtained before them by suffering a considerable loss. Good professional advice is essential here.

After these investments have been completed, there may well be more money available for investment as time goes by. There are firms which can give advice about the stock market, and it is advisable to use their services because dentists are so busy earning money in the dental surgery, they don't really have enough time to speculate; and amateurs invariably make mistakes. In many ventures hours can make all the difference in buying or selling, with regard to making a profit on a deal. This applies even to ordinary sober sounding shares as well as the high risk ventures. And there are many of the latter about. Almost anyone who has had some money to invest will have had his fingers burnt at some stage over some sure fire get-rich-quick deal, from pyramid parties via horse racing and the stock exchange to that little local business venture with the boys at the golf club. It's a sure bet that if none of us went in for these high risk investments then collectively we would all be a great deal better off in ten years' time. The golden rule with such high risk investments is not to put money into them unless you are prepared to lose it. Similarly you should never stretch your business finances so tight that you are relying on income from a big job to pay for day to day expenses, or get yourself in a position where you rely on a risky investment to get you out of trouble. If you cannot afford to lose money, do not put it at risk. (It is worth remarking at this point that the worst financial risk of all is going off with another woman. There is a terrible price to pay, since running two homes is expensive and the spurned wife will still need to be maintained. And the new association will be plagued by envy, because the new wife may well resent every alimony payment. Unless you can afford it, do not put your money or your happiness at risk.)

Health in the Practice

Financial health is of course all part of the health of a good practice. Cash flow is the lifeblood of any good business, but there is much more to it than that. If the basic business is not healthy then the cash flow will just not be there.

The health of your practice depends on the correct attitude of mind, just like everything else. You ought to have a philosophy of practice which is going to achieve what you want to achieve and this philosophy should be woven into the very material of your business. It is helpful to have your philosophy written down. If you cannot write it yourself, then use someone else's writing — use this if you wish. Take the relevant sections and ask your staff to read them regularly so that they keep up with your thinking and your ideals, and read it from time to time yourself to avoid becoming rusty. Ultimately it will be a great help for you to write something down (even if it is only a precis of something else) because writing will fix it in your own mind and clarify parts which you did not comprehend. It will also enable you to clarify any areas of disagreement.

The basis of practice health is love. And the most important person to direct that love towards is the patient. All things in the practice are done for the well being and comfort of the patient. Realise that he or she is an individual, unique in every way. Understand him, and encourage your staff to understand him also. We must all be 'people dentists'. Remember that love begets love. We all want to be loved and to love in return. This is a basic human trait, and is well developed in the most mature people. Since you will be coping more and more with mature people as your practice matures, you should always remember their need to be loved. Let them feel that they are in a family atmosphere at your practice. Never say unkind things about them behind their backs because this will also affect your thinking and your staff's thinking, and will be apparent in your attitude, and endeavour. Your staff must love the patients too and they should all be well aware of their responsibility to do so. The attitude starts at the top, and staff should take their example from you on this point; usually they are only too happy to, but occasionally you find someone who is uncooperative. In this case it is better to ask them to seek employment elsewhere, and the sooner the better.

The importance of staff relationships should never be underestimated, not only with the patients and the boss but also with each other. There are several things one can do to ensure that these relationships mature along the right lines and most of the ways are directly concerned with communication. The reason that the majority of marriages break up is lack of communication; for the same reason staff relationships sour. Opportunities must be provided somehow for individual staff to communicate with the boss, and other opportunities for them to communicate with each other. Time must be set aside occasionally for individual staff members to talk to the boss on a one-to-one basis, and this should be done in a situation permitting them to speak their minds freely, with no other person present to put a brake on what they want to say. People can speak their minds more easily in a relaxed atmosphere and it can be surprising what you learn about your own business, supplementary supplies, other staff members, etc. Staff may also make useful suggestions for improving aspects of the running the business where they have found snags. Sometimes these ideas will involve a change of duties for yourself or other members of your staff.

Continuity is another aspect of a healthy practice. It is important to try and keep your staff with you for long periods of time, as patients get to know them and relate to them, and this helps to build up the family atmosphere. Continuity comes easily when staff know they are appreciated and it is so important to show this appreciation in deeds as well as words. Do pay good wages. Happy staff who work willingly really earn them, and they are an investment, since good staff promote a happy and efficient business which promotes increased turnover. Give Christmas bonuses and take the trouble to write a little note of appreciation on their Christmas card. It may only be once a year but it does much to promote loyalty. Make sure you give something to show that you have remembered their birthday. A bottle of gin or bourbon might help their party along; or just knowing it is in the cupboard can be a great thing for some people. A few hours free time is also much appreciated especially when you are having an afternoon off to go to a study club or to play golf.

But it is not only positive things that must be considered, there are negative things that must be avoided. Never, never tell one member of the staff off in front of other staff or patients. Always ask them to see you later in private, and then be careful how you administer the reprimand. People are funny creatures. Start off with a compliment, then deliver the reprimand and then finish up by saying something nice again. It really is worth while. And don't forget to say thank you when they work through the lunch hour or stay late. People can be so loyal they make you feel humble, and in a good practice they will make tremendous sacrifices of time and effort in order to accommodate to difficulties. Let them see you appreciate it.

Finally, think of dental health. Your own dental health and your staff's dental health. Your own attitude of mind towards dentistry *is* the state of your own mouth. Have you had the sort of dentistry you are recommending to your patients? If not, why not? What right have you to suggest that they should have extensive dental treatment when you haven't bothered with it yourself? How do you imagine patients are going to react when they see that your receptionist or nurse badly needs dental treatment? or if it is obvious that you need the crowns just as badly as they do? It will be seen a sham. And so will your practice. I well remember one dentist who had his whole mouth rebuilt and commented afterwards that he looked upon it as an investment which he knew would pay off a hundred fold. This is indeed the other side of the coin and I hope it reflects your attitude of mind. So invest in health. Start with yourself and your own health, general and dental, and then your practice health and your financial health. You will not only be healthy but happy and wise as well as wealthy, and you will live to enjoy it too!

11

What To Do Now

Philosophising is all very well, but in itself, it does not achieve anything. You can read this work and many more like it and dream about it for years but get nowhere. That is the difference between the dreamer and the achiever. The achiever not only sees the possibilities for the future, he goes out and makes it happen. If you want to achieve anything in your life then you have to make a firm commitment NOW that you are going to be an achiever and not just a hearer of the word, and that you are going to be prepared to pay the price in study, work and discomfort. But even assuming that you are prepared to do whatever it takes in terms of effort, just how do you go about it? All right, so you accept that there is room for a reconstruction dental practice on every main street in the land, but how do you achieve it on yours? And how do you achieve the background happiness at home and completion of character growth necessary to produce fulfilment of your whole self; to become a self actualising person?

The necessary tools are absolute honesty in self discipline, patience, determination and a realisation that you are unique. With these tools you can first of all set out to master yourself. Then with growing knowledge of your own uniqueness you can plot your future.

Take Time

The first and most important thing to understand is that things take time. Rome wasn't built in a day. So do be patient and realistic, and above all, don't trample on your bread and butter in reaching out for the cake. The cake may be further away than you think and you will need the bread and butter to tide you over until you get there. It takes about five years to turn your practice over to three tier style dentistry. During this period you will have to maintain your class 3 patients in order to safeguard your income. Do try to educate them by dropping little verbal seeds which can be picked up in the future such as 'I hope you do the football pools/state lottery/premium bonds etc'. When they ask why you can say that you have big plans for their mouth. Many of them will let it drop for the present but bring it up again in six months or a year's time. Others will take it up straight away, and when they do you have the opening to educate them to their dental needs. This way they will become Class 2 patients and then missionaries for good dentistry. Patients they recommend will be expecting the four stage examination and a higher understanding of dental treatment, and so you collect the sort of patient you want. At the same time you can begin helping the type of patient you no longer want to find another dentist. This is not difficult, as most of them will realise that they do not fit in with your new image, and as your practice and fees gradually build up they will drift away of their own accord. Many such patients will leave your practice with great regret and will write a touching letter to which you should reply with love, wishing them well with their new dentist and assuring them that if ever

they need your services in the future you would be happy
to see them again. Should you be so booked up with Class 3
patients (which you are likely to be since everybody likes a
bargain) then you will have to do something about it or else
you will have no room for your new class one and two
people. Usually an increase in fees is the answer here, but
again it can be done with love, and people like to feel that
they have been considered and told something and not just
presented with a big bill. But do make sure that you don't
do this until you are ready. As you hasten slowly forward
with developing your practice, improving your decor and
staff attire etc., you will also need to be improving yourself.
So sit down and put a sheet of paper in front of you for self
analysis. Remember that you are going to think positively.
Firstly write down a list of faults or weaknesses in your
personal character. Then in an adjacent column write
down the positive virtue that you need to acquire in order
to overcome your weakness. For example, if you are always
forgetting things then write down that you are going to do
something to develop a good memory. If you are slipshod
then write that you want to develop application and
working for quality. If your mind is always wandering then
write that you want to develop your concentration. If you
are always starting things which you never finish, then
write down that you want perseverance. Now you have
done this you will want to know what to do to achieve the
positive virtues which you desire.

You have to 'reprogramme your computer,' write
something definite on your mental bit of paper, over and
over again so that it is difficult to rub out. So you say these
things every morning quietly like a litany, eg. I am a
persevering person and I always see things through. I do
have a good memory. I do carry out high class work and
apply all my skills and knowledge to the work in hand.

Repeat them every day at some quiet and private time. Make a determined commitment, it often helps to make a physical effort like clenching the hands and bracing all the muscles of the shoulders just to push the idea firmly into the mind. When you have done this look back upon what you have written and see if you have written down fear, or inadequate self image among your failings. If you have not then you had better add them to the list straight away because almost everybody has an inadequate self image. And the most overwhelming reason why we have an inadequate self image is fear. Fear is usually a buried factor, which has grown into the mind by conditioning when we were young. Such phrases as 'you'll never come to anything'. 'You are stupid! (clumsy, lazy, lying etc.)' breed a fear of failure and ridicule which is hard to shake off, and which stops one from sticking one's neck out and achieving things. Most of us never function at anything like our full capacity. Overcome your fears and doubts and be determined to acquire courage to go forward. Recondition your mind, reprogramme your computer for success. Determine that you are going to use your capacity to the full to achieve your goals. Say to yourself that you *are successful* and say it over and over again to yourself. Write it as the start of the list or litany of reprogramming points that you are going to keep quietly to yourself, but which you can repeat to yourself every day. In the meantime, think about your goals and write them down. Think hard, and think positive, think so hard that you can actually visualise your goal in your own mind, and visualise it in detail in glorious technicolour. This is a very important first step in turning your goal into a reality. Success depends on two things, having well defined goals, and being determined and effective in pursuit of them. These things are even more important than inborn ability.

Now think about your positive attributes. These are the foundations upon which you are going to build your success. Even if you do not think you have them as fully as your neighbour, it does not matter. You are going to succeed by using your assets to the full. Most people do not, and it is surprising how little extra effort is necessary to succeed. An average of one stroke less per round over a year is the difference between the top earning golf pro and an also ran! Five percent extra effort can make you into a winner. So make a list of your positive attributes and determine to improve them.

Now look back over your lists, and in particular your goals. Is it comprehensive enough? — or is it only half complete? Because if you do not know where you are going you are hardly likely to get there. It is not good enough just to say that you want to get somewhere in life because getting 'somewhere' leads nowhere. Be definite. And remember that your cross should be in balance. Avoid goals that are mutually contradictory. Do realise that you should have goals for your home and family as well as your business. Work, play, love and worship should all be represented. Anyone who has been to the Pankey Institute will be familiar with the sheets of paper they provide for writing down of one's goals. They include achievements (play the guitar, ride a horse, paint a picture etc.) travel, what you want to see, what knowledge you want to acquire, what you want to earn and what you want to own. The sheets end up with one called 'what I want out of life' which is a summary of all one's desires. This is a good point to look back and re-examine what one has written.

Does it all really fit in with your character and unique personality? Does it really conform to the type of person you want to be? Do you really want this or is it that you just want to keep up with Jones? Can you make your aspirations effective or are they too grand to be achievable? Or so small as to be hardly worth the effort?

Are your goals all positively expressed? Remember that recognising your faults is only the first step to eradicating them. That is the positive thing, acquiring the improvement your desire. Avoid the trap of making your goals into limitations. What the mind can conceive and believe, it can achieve, so make sure that your goals stretch you. Aim for the top in all things, think positive and believe in yourself.

There should always be a time scale to your goals. Some goals can be attained in months, others take years. It is not only governments that can have five year plans. So keep your list of goals somewhere safe and take it out from time to time and appraise how you are getting on.

If you are not proceeding as well as you expected, then analyse why, and do something about it. Perhaps a change in economic conditions made your goal unreasonable. Remember, things do happen outside our control. The fact that you may have to modify your goals because of external factors does not matter. You may decide in any case that you do not really want to achieve a certain goal after all. This is all for you to decide. You are the captain, and your ship should go in the direction you want even if you do have to weather a few storms on the way.

I hope these words have been useful, and helpful. The basic philosophy has been extremely useful to me in my life and I hope it will help others to find joy and peace and fulfilment. Go and hear others talking about it over and over again and in particular don't miss the opportunity to hear L.D. Pankey or Loren Miller. And try and make friends with others who think the same way and strive for the same ideals, so you can help each other towards a deeper understanding. This way you will hear more as you listen, until eventually you own the philosophy for your-self. Then, like me, you will say thank you to L.D. and thank you Loren for a gift more valuable than almost anything else in the world.

Recommended Reading

1 *Evaluation Diagnosis and Treatment of Occlusal Problems*, Peter E. Dawson (Mosby).

2 *The Third Force*, Frank Gable (Thomas Jefferson Research Centre, Pasadena, California). Abraham Maslow is difficult reading in the original. This synopsis of his work is useful.

3 *Occlusal Equilibration and Temporomandibular Joint Dysfunction*, Nathan Allen Shore (Lippincott Co., Philadelphia, Pennsylvania).

4 *Occlusion*, Ramfjord & Ash (W. B. Saunders Co., Philadelphia, Pennsylvania).

5 *Personalised Denture Proceedures*, Earl Pound (Denar Corp., Anaheim, California).

6 *Atlas of Occlusal Analysis*, Arne G. Lauritzen (HAH Publications, Colorado Springs, Colorado).

7 *As A Man Thinketh*, James Allen (Fleming J. Revell Company, Old Tappau, New Jersey).

8 *Comments on the Use of Nickel and Amalgum in Dentistry*, David Egglestone (Newport Beach, California).

9 *Simple Thoughts on Science of Thought*, Henry Thomas Hamblin (Science of Thought Press Ltd, Chichester, Sussex).

10 *A Pocket Popper*, David Miller.

11 The Nexus Group Inc., Cave Creek, Arizona.